Evaluating Worksite Health Promotion

David H. Chenoweth, PhD, FAWHP
East Carolina University
President, Health Management Associates

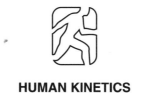

HUMAN KINETICS

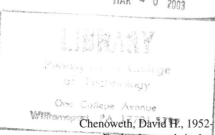
Library of Congress Cataloging-in-Publication Data

Chenoweth, David H., 1952-
    Evaluating worksite health promotion / David H. Chenoweth.
        p. cm.
    Includes bibliographical references and index.
    ISBN 0-7360-3647-4
        1. Health promotion. 2. Worksite health promotion. 3. Employee health promotion. I.
    Title.

    RC969.H43 C475 2001
    658.3'82--dc21   2001039616

ISBN: 0-7360-3647-4

Acquisitions Editor: Amy N. Clocksin; **Developmental Editor and Writer:** Elaine Mustain; **Assistant Editors:** Maggie Schwarzentraub, Lee Alexander; **Copyeditor:** Scott Weckerly; **Proofreader:** Red Inc.; **Indexer:** Craig Brown; **Permission Manager:** Dalene Reeder; **Graphic Designer:** Nancy Rasmus; **Graphic Artist:** Yvonne Griffith; **Cover Designer:** Keith Blomberg; **Photographer (cover):** Tom Roberts; **Photographer (interior):** Leslie A. Woodrum; **Art Managers:** Craig Newsom, Carl Johnson; **Illustrator:** Tom Roberts; **Printer:** Sheridan

Printed in the United States of America   10 9 8 7 6 5 4 3 2 1

Human Kinetics
Web site: www.humankinetics.com
United States: Human Kinetics
P.O. Box 5076
Champaign, IL 61825-5076
800-747-4457
e-mail: humank@hkusa.com

Canada: Human Kinetics
475 Devonshire Road Unit 100
Windsor, ON N8Y 2L5
800-465-7301 (in Canada only)
e-mail: orders@hkcanada.com

Europe: Human Kinetics
Units C2/C3 Wira Business Park
West Park Ring Road
Leeds LS16 6EB, United Kingdom
+44 (0) 113 278 1708
e-mail: hk@hkeurope.com

Australia: Human Kinetics
57A Price Avenue
Lower Mitcham, South Australia 5062
08 8277 1555
e-mail: liahka@senet.com.au

New Zealand: Human Kinetics
P.O. Box 105-231, Auckland Central
09-523-3462
e-mail: hkp@ihug.co.nz

To Nellie M. Blizzard and Donald R. Farthing Sr., who taught me the essence of preparation, discipline, perseverance, and humility.

Contents

Preface   vii

Acknowledgments   ix

Part I   Foundations of Evaluation

Chapter 1   **Introduction to Worksite Health Promotion Evaluation**   **3**

What Is Evaluation?   4

Purpose of Evaluation   4

Categorizing Evaluation   6

Chapter 2   **Basic Evaluation Procedures**   **13**

Working With Variables   14

Working With Groups for Comparison   26

Working With Experimental and Non-Experimental Designs   28

Working With Data   33

Part II   Instruments of Analysis

Chapter 3   **Project Effectiveness Analysis**   **51**

Claims Data Analysis   52

Risk Factor Cost Appraisal   72

Chapter 4   **Financial Analysis**   **79**

Forecasting   81

Break-Even Analysis   104

Cost-Effectiveness Analysis   110

Benefit-Cost Analysis   118

Part III   Planning, Conducting, and Presenting Evaluations

Chapter 5   **Planning and Conducting Evaluations**   **133**

Step One: Establish Goals   135

Step Two: Identify Evaluation Resources   146

Step Three: Define Scope and Specificity   148

Step Four: Select an Evaluation Design   155

Step Five: Manage Data   158

Chapter 6   **Preparing and Presenting Evaluation Results**   **171**

Interpreting Results   172

Identifying Stakeholders and Their Needs   177

Reporting Evaluation Results   179

Applying Evaluation Results   186

Appendix   189

Bibliography   193

Index   195

About the Author   205

Preface

All social institutions or subsystems, whether medical, educational, religious, economic, or political, are required to provide proof of their legitimacy and effectiveness in order to justify society's continued support. Both the demand for and the type of acceptable proof will depend largely on the nature of the relationship between the social institution and the public. In general, a balance will be struck between faith and fact, reflecting the degree of man's respect for authority and tradition within the particular system versus his skepticism and desire for tangible proof of work.

Edward Suchman, 1967

Here Suchman reminds us that any intervention needs to be scrutinized to determine its real value. But many of today's health promotion management personnel do not have the skills they need to perform a credible evaluation of their programs. When this deficit is present, it is usually due to an academic background that failed to provide the financial and management skills or the measurement and statistical expertise needed for objective program evaluation. This book provides such professionals with the information they need to develop both, as well as serving as a text for new evaluation courses that are now being developed to fill the earlier void in worksite health promotion (WHP) curricula.

Written for both students and practitioners, this book provides step-by-step models for creating a sound evaluation plan, assessing the availability and need for specific resources, and designing and implementing an appropriate evaluation tailored to your needs. Part I provides you with an introduction to evaluation and the value of doing a quality evaluation. Chapter 1 defines key concepts such as measurement, analysis, and evaluation, as well as defining distinctions between process, impact, and outcome-based evaluation. Chapter 2 discusses fundamental concepts and techniques involved in working with experimental groups and designs, data, and variables.

Part II contains two chapters that highlight analytical instruments used in WHP evaluation. Chapter 3 highlights claims data analysis (CDA) and risk factor cost appraisal, and how such information can be used in program evaluations. It also provides information on how to design instruments for gathering qualitative data and how to analyze those data. Chapter 4 highlights various tools of econometric analysis including cost-effectiveness analysis, break-even analysis, forecasting, and benefit-cost analysis. Factors that threaten the validity and reliability of an evaluation are also identified.

Part III consists of two chapters that focus on planning, conducting, and presenting evaluation outcome data. In addition, tips are offered for ensuring quality control and preparing an evaluation presentation tailored to specific audiences. Chapter 5 offers worksite-tested tips on setting goals and objectives, how to assess on-site (organizational) versus off-site (public and commercial) resources, selecting an evaluation design and the outcome variables to measure, how to request appropriate data, and determining a reasonable time frame for conducting an evaluation. Chapter 6 presents a worksite-tested process for identifying stakeholders and interpreting data for consideration in a presentation. Insights are also given for applying evaluation results in a worksite setting.

Review questions appear at the end of every section or two within the chapters, rather than at the end of each chapter. This is particularly useful in the longer chapters, as it prompts students to review at practical intervals, reinforcing information to provide a solid foundation for what follows. Multiple case studies in each chapter illustrate how to apply the material in practical settings, and computer tips advise the reader on how to use technology to enhance evaluation efforts. *What Would You Do?* scenarios at the end of each chapter require students to devise plans of action to address problem situations. Key terms are in bold when they are first introduced in the text. Readers of all levels, then, can take advantage of whichever tools are most appropriate for themselves.

Whether you are a college student preparing for a career in an organizational health promotion capacity or a seasoned practitioner interested in measuring the impact of your health promotion efforts, I hope you'll find this book a valuable resource for enhancing your evaluation efforts.

Acknowledgments

Over the past two decades, I have had the pleasure of working with many organizations and their talented WHP personnel on various evaluation projects. Many of these organizations are referenced, directly and indirectly, throughout this book. These organizations—from North Carolina to California—deserve a hearty thank-you for the opportunity they have afforded me to hone and apply my skills over the years. Finally, I extend a great deal of personal gratitude to Elaine Mustain, my project editor at Human Kinetics, for her vast knowledge, insight, and professionalism in keeping me on track through the lengthy process of writing this book.

PART I

Foundations of Evaluation

Introduction to Worksite Health Promotion Evaluation

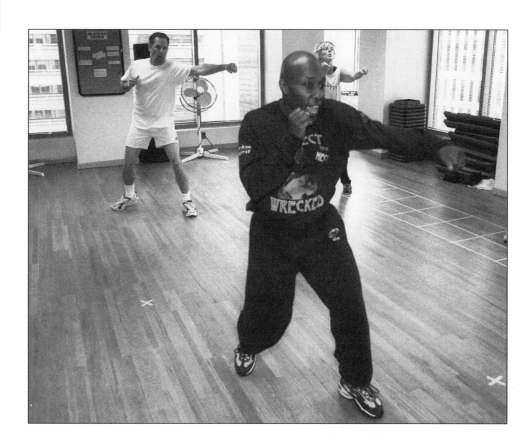

After reading this chapter and answering the questions at the end, you should be able to do the following:

- List several reasons why evaluation should be a part of all programs.

- Describe three ways to categorize evaluation.

- Distinguish and describe process, impact, and outcome evaluation.

- Determine the appropriate types of evaluation to use when measuring qualitative versus quantitative aspects of a program evaluation.

- Distinguish between various types of periodic review evaluations.

Early supporters of health promotion activities in the worksite setting were committed to health promotion and disease-prevention efforts because they just made sense. The time for blind acceptance of health promotion's effectiveness, however, has passed. Programs that had foregone evaluation in favor of investing in activities are now in trouble. At present, corporate leaders are asking for data to support the continuation of long-standing and, in certain cases, expensive programs. Other organizations, now establishing new programs, are setting clear expectations for measurable results. The measurement and evaluation of program outcomes has thus become a crucial activity in organizational health-promotion programming.

What Is Evaluation?

Imagine the following situations:

- While doing a health promotion internship at a large worksite, a college senior is asked by his supervisor to determine if the newly purchased medical self-care manual is cost-effective.
- In the first month of a new job at a managed care organization, the claims data analyst is approached by her boss, who asks her if she can calculate the economic cost of smoking for a corporate client.
- On the eve of his 21st year with the health care organization, the human resources director has been asked to implement an integrated health data management system and to track its impact on occupational injuries.

What do all of these situations have in common? A need to conduct an appropriate evaluation: to determine the amount or worth of something.

Whether you are a student preparing for a career in worksite health promotion (WHP), the youngest employee on a health management staff, or a seasoned professional embarking on a comprehensive evaluation project, it is important to understand what evaluation is, why evaluation should be conducted, what the evaluation process comprises, and how decision makers can benefit from a properly conducted evaluation.

REVIEW QUESTIONS: DEFINITION OF EVALUATION

1. What is meant by *proof of their legitimacy and effectiveness* in Suchman's quote in the preface?
2. What are several reasons for conducting a program evaluation?

Purpose of Evaluation

Evaluation enhances decision making because it provides accurate information for determining the impact of health-promotion programs. For instance, evaluation can help a program planner determine whether participants were satisfied with a low back program, if a medical self-care workshop reduced unnecessary health care visits, or whether an exercise facility should be expanded. Without reliable evaluation data, it is impossible to make such decisions based on anything but assumptions and intuition.

There are many aspects of evaluating a program's effectiveness, including the following:

- **Appraising progress:** An evaluation can help determine whether a program is moving in the right direction and is likely to achieve its goal. For example, is a three-month-old program approximately halfway toward achieving its six-month goal?

- **Comparing different programs:** Programs can be compared with one another to determine which are the most effective in reaching specific goals. For example, benefit-cost analysis, break-even analysis, and cost-effectiveness analysis (see chapter 4) can be used to examine two or more programs simultaneously (e.g., low back versus smoking cessation) or to compare two or more versions of a similar program (e.g., low back stretching versus low back lifting techniques).

- **Complying with funding specifications:** Grant-funded and other externally financed evaluations typically require formal evaluations to determine whether the goals and objectives have been met; if the program is cost-effective; and whether the program should be continued, expanded, or discontinued.

- **Determining end-of-program outcomes:** As the program comes to an official end, an evaluation can provide information on how well the final results fulfilled the initial goals.

- **Informing key groups about the program:** The basic thrust of a well-designed and well-implemented process is to provide systematic feedback about health-promotion programs and activities to management, staff, and participants.

Counting the Cost

An accurate evaluation can provide valuable feedback to decision makers on whether certain worksite interventions are working. For instance, a health care organization had established a hotline for high-risk employees to receive biweekly tips on how to comply with their personalized risk-reduction programs. The organization tracked the monthly costs of the program intervention, the participation, and the compliance rates throughout the six months of intervention. Outcome data indicated several unfavorable findings:

- Participation dropped nearly 50% midway in the program.
- Self-reported compliance rates dropped nearly 50%.
- Risk factor costs dropped only 5%.

The figures showed that the cost of implementing the program exceeded the cost-savings by nearly a five-to-one ratio. Based on these facts, the organization decided to replace the hotline program with an on-site risk-reduction program that produced a favorable benefit-to-cost ratio within its first six months of operation. The initial evaluation provided timely feedback to the organization and revealed the ineffectiveness of a particular intervention; thus, it generated the impetus for a more cost-effective intervention.

REVIEW QUESTIONS: PURPOSE OF EVALUATION

1. What are several aspects of evaluating a program's effectivness?
2. How can an evaluation enhance decision making?

Categorizing Evaluation

There are many approaches one could take to categorizing evaluation. For example, one could organize evaluation according to qualitative versus quantitative issues, to the use of results, or to the timing of the evaluation.

Qualitative Versus Quantitative Issues

According to this way of organizing evaluations, there are only two basic types:

- **Project effectiveness evaluation (qualitative).** This type assesses how a program can be improved before or during implementation and how it affects quality of life and health issues. This kind of evaluation answers the question, *Is this program effective? If so, what makes it successful? If not, why not? How can it be improved?*

- **Financial evaluation (quantitative).** This type answers questions about the financial costs, benefits, and feasibility of programs. It provides information necessary for deciding what programs can be afforded, how to adjust programs for affordability, and whether to discontinue or retain certain programs.

Use of Information

Another way of approaching evaluation is to consider how the information will be used. Two systems of categorization have been developed for this approach:

1. The **process/impact/outcome system**
2. The **formative/summative system**

Both of these systems think of evaluation according to how the information will be used. Formative evaluation, for example, focuses on assessing how programs can be improved as they progress. Summative evaluation analyzes a program at its conclusion to see what has been accomplished. It determines whether the program should continue, and if so, how it should be changed. The author prefers the process/impact/outcome system, however, because it enables one to make further distinctions in postprogram evaluation types. Thus, this text illustrates and explains the process/impact/outcome system rather than the formative/summative categories.

Process Evaluation

Process evaluation provides information during program implementation on what improvements could be made. It can focus on either qualitative or quantitative questions.

Qualitative issues would include aspects of program delivery such as program registration, educational content, and instructor effectiveness. For example, by looking at the age, gender, and job category of employees who have participated in the various program offerings, the evaluator could assess whether one delivery mode, teaching method, or incentive appears to have drawn certain segments of the workforce more effectively than another. Reactions from participants about programming schedules, fitness center hours, or workshop speakers could show program administrators what changes

---

Computer Tip

When reviewing program management software, check to see that the features fit your needs. For example, specific features requested by many WHP personnel include the following:

- Communications—personalized home pages, instant access to e-mail addresses, staff-only news area
- Participant services—activity logging, medical questionnaire, personal bank accounts that track activity credits
- Tools for retention—fitness assessments, incentive programs, gated access (so only medically-cleared employees can see the entire site)
- Facility management—inventory management, personnel assignments, budgetary cash flow

The key is to identify your needs first to see how various software programs mesh with your personnel and your organization's evaluation goals. Finally, request either a demonstration of the software or a trial version of the software.

might be necessary to improve participation rates. The tools of qualitative analysis include short questionnaires, verbal solicitation, focus groups, suggestion boxes, e-mail communications, and other on-site media.

Financial issues can also be addressed by process evaluation. Predicting when the break-even point will be, how much the cost-savings will be, and how long until they are realized can tell program administrators whether they should scale back or expand their original plans. The tools for making these kinds of financial predictions are discussed in detail in chapter 4.

Impact Evaluation

As the intermediate strategy, **impact evaluation** assesses the overall effectiveness of a program in producing desirable levels of knowledge, attitudes, behaviors, health status, or skills in a target population. For example, how many people stopped smoking? How many people can effectively perform CPR? How much do people know about AIDS? Overall, behavioral, attitudinal, and cultural changes that occur during an intervention are measured by impact evaluation using one or more survey techniques to compare pre- and postprogram changes. Common evaluation tools include

- questionnaires,
- health risk appraisals,
- health care claims data reports,
- occupational injury reports,
- absenteeism data,
- culture audits (i.e., observing the worksite environment), and
- productivity/quality reports.

Impact evaluation measures the degree of change resulting from the program. An example would be to look at the nutritional habits of employees before the start of a program, then use the same survey at the end of the program. The survey could assess the degree to which employees made positive nutritional changes and how these changes may have affected the corporate culture (e.g., more employees ate healthier snacks at break time).

Although impact evaluation can provide evaluators with specific types of quantitative feedback within a particular intervention, this intermediate-level evaluation is merely a prerequisite for the bottom-line results that can be determined from outcome evaluation.

Outcome Evaluation

Considered the back-end strategy along the evaluation continuum, **outcome evaluation** determines and quantifies cost-savings that may occur when an intervention affects absenteeism, productivity, health care utilization, and the like. Outcome evaluation focuses on the question, *Did the intervention cause the changes that occurred, and if so, was the financial cost feasible?* For example, did the intervention do any of the following:

- Reduce the average blood pressure and medication usage following a hypertension reduction program, thus lowering prescription costs?
- Drop the prevalence of stress-related disorders requiring counseling interventions after an employee assistance program?
- Drop the level of miscommunication between benefits and employee health and safety personnel after an integrated data management system was established, increasing efficiency and lowering the cost of company administration?

- Reduce the number of work-related injuries after a risk identification program, reducing the cost of workers' compensation?
- Decrease low back pain incidence after a healthy-back awareness program, reducing the number of doctor's visits, and thus decreasing the cost of insurance?
- Drop the demand for requested health care services from the occupational health nurse?
- Create enough savings to cover the cost of the intervention?

The instruments of outcome evaluation include claims data analysis, cost-effectiveness analysis, and benefit-cost analysis. These techniques are discussed in chapters 3 and 4.

Note that in nonmedical fields of evaluation, the terms *impact* and *outcome* are sometimes used in reverse: Outcome refers to the more immediate effects of programs, methods, or professional activity; impact refers to the distant or ultimate effects of social programs. The usage in this text reflects the established meanings of these terms in biomedical and health services research. They refer to impacts as physiological changes and to outcomes as consequences of impacts in terms of quality of life and economic benefits.

Timing of Evaluation

The categories of evaluation that depend on its timing are

- periodic reviews and
- longitudinal data analysis.

Periodic Reviews

Multiple evaluations conducted within a particular time frame are known as **periodic reviews** because they are used to assess various performance measures at designated intervals. Common types of periodic reviews are

- quality assurance,
- monthly reviews,
- quarterly and semiannual reviews, and
- annual reviews.

Quality Assurance

Today's quality assurance initiatives, such as **total quality management** (TQM) and **continuous quality improvement** (CQI), were introduced in many American worksites over 50 years ago. Initially, TQM and CQI standards were developed primarily to identify manufacturing quagmires tied to product design and assembly-line operations. Eventually, quality assurance measures were applied to service units as well, and in the 1980s, they were extended to worksite health promotion programs. Examples of operating standards may include the following:

- The fitness center is opened and closed promptly at designated times.
- Fitness center equipment is cleaned several times per week.
- Fitness center equipment malfunctions are repaired within 24 hours of breakdown.
- Staff members consistently greet all employees and display strong customer-oriented skills.

- Employee medical data are accessible and managed only by certified medical personnel.
- Instructors' teaching methods adhere to organizational standards.
- All health screenings are conducted only by certified technicians in a confidential manner to protect each employee's privacy.
- All printed and electronic materials are approved by the program director before dissemination.
- All ergonomic enhancements comply with standards set by the Occupational Safety and Health Administration (OSHA).

Measuring employee satisfaction is a very important aspect of any organization's quality assurance program. These efforts can generate important information for staff members to review in determining where and how well they are meeting customers' needs and interests. Although the scope of employee satisfaction is quite broad, some common areas include the following:

- How participants view the quality of the health management staff
- The quality of current program offerings
- Privacy and confidentiality safeguards for managing medical and health status data
- The level of sensitivity and responsiveness of hotline counselors
- The value of participation incentives

Quality assurance measures can also relate to performance standards established for staff members. To illustrate, consider the following questions:

- Are staff members maintaining their professional certification by earning adequate continuing education units (CEUs)?
- Does each staff member clearly subscribe to the industry's code of ethics?
- Are program instructors generating high participation in their activities?

Monthly, Quarterly, Semiannual, and Annual Reviews

Monthly reviews identify, track, and summarize daily and weekly statistics, all of which can ultimately be converted into a monthly record. Monthly reviews are appropriate on other performance measures ranging from budgetary assessments to participation levels in health promotion interventions and changes in employee health status. For example, monthly reviews can track a department's cash flow, thereby helping decision makers understand how fixed and variable expense items vary from month to month. Monthly reviews of risk factor prevalence rates can provide valuable information to staff members on which risk-reduction activities are most effective in reducing targeted risk factors.

Quarterly and semiannual reviews encompass several months of data and therefore are more reliable instruments than monthly assessments in detecting trends. They are especially useful for analyzing the effectiveness of an organization's program mix. For example, assume an organization has an on-site fitness center that has operated year-round for the past 10 years and offers a myriad of aerobic and strength training programs. Staff members recently expanded the scope of the current programs by adding a strength and flexibility program for the low back. The new program was implemented midyear and was set to be evaluated at quarterly and semiannual intervals. These periodic reviews can provide staff members with timely feedback on the following:

- Whether the low back program is generating more fitness center participation
- What types of people who initially participate in the low back program eventually move on to other fitness center programs—for example, by gender, age range, occupation, and so on
- Whether the program is reducing the number of low back injuries in a timely manner

Quarterly and semiannual reviews are also particularly valuable for evaluating short-term programs. For instance, an organization may offer on-site *lunch-'n'-learn* seminars for eight weeks with the goal of improving employee dietary habits. Participants complete weekly dietary intake logs that are then reviewed at the end of the first and second months. With this feedback, decision makers can determine if participants are making any positive changes during the program. However, by adding a semiannual review of participants' dietary habits, decision makers can determine if any initial changes were maintained, thus determining the need to offer a future lunch-'n'-learn seminar.

The final type of periodic review is an annual review, comprising monthly, quarterly, and semiannual reviews. These reviews allow staff to determine if an intervention's initial and short-term impact is intensifying, fading, or unchanged.

Summary of WHP Evaluation Categories

1. Quality versus quantity

- **Project effectiveness evaluation (quality)** assesses how a program can be improved before or during implementation, and its effects on quality of life and health issues.
- **Financial evaluation (quantity)** answers questions about the financial costs, benefits, and feasibility of programs.

2. Use of information

- Process
- Impact
- Outcome evaluation

Samples of the types of factors addressed by process, impact, and outcome evaluations:

Process	Impact	Outcome
Financial incentives	Blood pressure control	Number of doctor visits
Participant opinions	Diabetes management	Absenteeism
Educational content	Consumer attitudes	Productivity
Instructor competency	Smoking cessation	Employer-employee relations
Timing of financial break-even point		Cost of benefits
Predicted cost-savings		

3. Timing of evaluation

- **Periodic reviews** can be monthly, quarterly, semiannual, or annual.
- **Longitudinal data analysis** examines data from a several-year span.

Longitudinal Data Analysis

Longitudinal data analysis involves monitoring and evaluating data over a multiyear time frame. Longitudinal data analyses are appropriate for tracking program participation and health and behavior change outcomes over time, as well as long-term financial analyses such as benefit-cost analysis (chapter 4).

REVIEW QUESTIONS: CATEGORIZING EVALUATION

1. Name and define three ways of categorizing evaluation. Name the types of evaluation that make up each of the three.
2. Distinguish among process, impact, and outcome evaluations by giving examples of each.
3. What kinds of program quality questions are relevant to process evaluation?
4. What type of evaluation is directed toward measuring qualitative aspects of program delivery such as participation, educational content, and instructor competency?
5. What types of evaluation tools can be used to compare pre-intervention states with postintervention changes?
6. What factor primarily distinguishes process, impact, and outcome evaluations from one another?

CHAPTER REVIEW

Summary

Today's cost-conscious economy has made accurate program evaluation more crucial than ever as the number of worksite health promotion programs continues to grow. Well-designed evaluations can provide program planners with a clear-cut structure to determine the effectiveness of specific interventions as well as their costs and benefits. Evaluations can be categorized in at least three ways. First, they can be organized by qualitative versus quantitative issues to determine how a program can be improved and how costs and benefits can be compared. Second, they can be organized by the use of results, as in process, impact, and outcome evaluations. Finally, they can be categorized by evaluation chronology—that is, when the evaluation will be conducted. Periodic reviews and longitudinal data analyses make up this type of evaluation. Chapter 2 explains how to understand evaluation designs, how to tailor interventions for appropriate evaluation, and how to work with variables, groups, and data.

What Would You Do?

You have recently been hired in an entry-level health promotion position at a large managed care organization (MCO). In addition to providing health care services to 100 local employers, the MCO provides on-site health promotion programs to approximately 20% of this population. Your immediate supervisor has asked you to determine the level of client satisfaction with these health promotion programs. A few days later, the president of the MCO asks your supervisor for some hard numbers to show the programs' effectiveness. With the assumption that the data will be supportive, they are to be shared with the marketing department to use in renegotiating future contracts with existing clients. What type or types of evaluations will you propose? Justify your answer.

2 Basic Evaluation Procedures

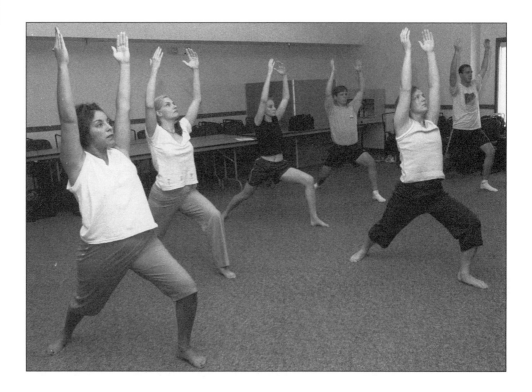

After reading this chapter and answering the questions at the end, you should be able to do the following:

- Define the three types of variables in worksite health promotion.
- Explain simple versus complex variables and objective versus subjective variables.
- Discuss tips on how to use at least three specific variables.
- Differentiate among experimental, control, and comparison groups.
- Compare and contrast the major types of evaluation designs.
- List major considerations in selecting an evaluation design.
- Compare and contrast quantitative and qualitative data.
- Identify the threats to internal and external validity and explain how an appropriate evaluation design can enhance control.
- Discuss how to design valid instruments for gathering qualitative data.
- Discuss how to analyze qualitative data.

Before you can use the tools of analysis in WHP evaluation, you must acquire a basic understanding of variables, designs, and data, and how to work with them to increase your chances of reaching valid conclusions.

Working With Variables

There are three types of variables in worksite health promotion: independent, dependent, and confounding.

- **Independent variables** are the interventions that program planners think will make an impact, such as an exercise facility, brochures on medical self-help, or a free program on smoking cessation. The interventions that are developed (and are therefore necessary to evaluate) will be the givens, or independent variables, in your evaluation.

- **Dependent variables** are the factors those interventions are seeking to affect, such as blood pressure, body composition, stress levels, or exercise habits. When properly written, dependent variables will represent the measurable and quantifiable aspects of each intervention's goal.

- **Confounding variables** are those factors that could interfere with the effect of the intervention and its intended outcome. Here are several examples of confounding variables:

    - Budgetary pitfalls—Senior management may decide to reduce the health management budget to free up money for other business operations; in addition, a decline in participant fees may inhibit the continuation or quality of a program.

    - Inclement weather—Poor weather conditions can hinder participation in an outdoor activity such as a lunchtime walking program.

    - Tough business climate—Growing competition in the marketplace may prompt employees to work longer hours and, in turn, sacrifice personal health-enhancement time.

    - Personnel competencies—Newly hired health management staff members may be less qualified than former staff members to sustain the momentum of the intervention.

    - Change in source of support—Key supporters may leave the company and be replaced by decision makers who are not philosophically supportive of the program.

    - Changing policies—Increasing participation fees or changing programming schedules may keep some employees, including high-risk individuals, from participating in certain programs.

    - Self-selection bias—Most worksite health promotion programs attract employees who voluntarily choose to participate in them. By volunteering to participate in a program intervention, employees have self-selected themselves. Participants tend to have more interest in their health than nonparticipants and, consequently, are more likely to participate in an intervention. Moreover, since most worksite health evaluations do not include a matched control group (nonparticipants), it is difficult to determine if any positive outcomes associated with a particular intervention are actually due to the intervention or this self-selection bias.

Confounding variables pose a serious threat to evaluators because they compromise the potential impact that an intervention can have on dependent variables, yet they are sometimes so difficult to spot that their effect may be attributed to the wrong cause. Confounding variables are often difficult to predict, much less control, and should be considered in every program evaluation. When a confounding variable appears in the midst of a program, evaluators must be sure to make note of it so it can be taken into account when the time comes for program evaluation.

Independent, dependent, and confounding variables may be further classified as simple versus complex variables and subjective versus objective variables. These subclassifications are discussed next, as well as tips on working with selected variables. How to identify and choose appropriate variables for a specific evaluation is discussed in chapter 5.

Simple Versus Complex Variables

Simple variables are relatively easy to define, measure, and quantify in a program evaluation while **complex variables** are multidimensional and, thus, require more effort. Several examples of each variable include the following:

Simple	Complex
• Aerobic capacity	• Absenteeism
• Blood pressure	• Diet management
• Body-fat percentage	• Health care cost management
• Flexibility	• Health care utilization control
• On-the-job injuries	• Productivity
• Smoking status	• Turnover

Simple variables can be measured with standardized protocols that have been established by a group of qualified scientists or by a professional organization. For instance, the most accurate way to measure a person's body fat is to use the hydrostatic (underwater) method, which is based on years of clinical research in various settings. Complex variables, on the other hand, cannot usually be measured by standardized, scientifically established methods, and they will usually be affected by a wide array of factors. For instance, suppose evaluators wish to use diet management as a measurement variable. Because this is a complex variable, they must make the following considerations:

- Understand that many things influence a person's diet, such as culture, genetics, values, environment, and age. Evaluators should take these factors into account when they design programs intended to influence diet management. If they wish to evaluate these programs reliably, they must be able to isolate the aspect of the program that is intended to affect the factor that influences diet.

- Establish a quantifiable goal to determine the level of success. For example, *Daily caloric intake will not exceed 2,500 calories and will not be composed of more than 30% fat.*

- Have a valid (accurate) tool to measure the quantifiable reference they have established—in this case, daily caloric intake.

Evaluators should recognize the differences between the simple versus complex variables and must handle each type with appropriate methods.

Objective Versus Subjective Variables

Objective variables differ from subjective variables in at least two respects: definition and measurement. **Objective variables** feature universally accepted definitions, measured by universally accepted methods that will result in universally accepted results. *Universally,* in this context, means *including everyone who is involved in the discussion or the effort in which the term is being used.* **Subjective variables** may be defined by a person's opinions or feelings; hence, they cannot be universally measured so that everyone will agree on the results.

To put it another way, if everyone who is using a variable in a specific context (or universe) agrees on what it means and how it is being measured, the variable is objective in that setting. If they do not, the variable is not objective in that setting. For example, suppose that one staff member has the power to define **absenteeism** as any absence from scheduled work hours. This definition is made known to everyone, and all evaluation efforts are based on it. Although this definition is not particularly useful (since it doesn't differentiate between scheduled and unscheduled absences, so very few significant conclusions could be based on it) this situation would demonstrate an objective use of the variable absenteeism. If everyone in the company is using the definition in all measurements and discussions of absenteeism, the definition is objective, relative to that company.

If, on the other hand, no one talks about what absenteeism means, it is entirely possible that the staff member who designs the program, the one who measures the program, and the management person who hears the results of the program will all use different definitions. These people could discuss their concept of absenteeism frequently without ever realizing that each of the others is talking about something quite different. Absenteeism has thus become a subjective variable. This subjective use of the variable absenteeism will result in meaningless evaluation because, unknown to one another, the staff are comparing apples to oranges to bananas.

Or consider a slightly different version of this scenario: Management has agreed on one definition of absenteeism, the WHP staff have all agreed on a second definition, and the workers who are participating in the program have never even considered that absenteeism could have a definition different from what each one has always assumed the term means. Even though two of these definitions have been agreed on by large groups of people, none of them is objective. The problem is that the individual workers and the two groups are all involved in the same universe (i.e., the WHP program for that company), but have not all agreed together on what they mean when they say absenteeism or on how the variable is being measured.

Measuring an objective variable correctly will yield valid (accurate) and reliable (consistent) results. Measuring an objective variable subjectively will yield invalid and unreliable results. Measuring a subjective variable will yield invalid and unreliable results no matter how it is done since no one is clear on what was being measured in the first place. The accuracy of measurements of an objective variable depends on

- the quality of the measurement tool,
- the quality of the measurement process, and
- the frequency of the measurement.

For example, when measuring blood pressure, evaluators should use a properly calibrated sphygmomanometer (cuff) and stethoscope to detect the presence of hypertension. Assuming these measurement tools are properly administered, a single blood pressure reading is not always indicative of a person's real blood pressure. Thus, several readings are typically performed to determine an average blood pressure. Thus, the accuracy of measurement increases as the quality and frequency of measurement increases.

As another example, suppose a supervisor ranks an employee's work performance as excellent, based solely on a visual observation of the worker's physical effort. Yet, several coworkers rank the employee's performance as good or average. Why the discrepancy? The employee's performance was ranked differently by the supervisor and coworkers because there was little, if any, objectivity in how productivity was measured. Yet it is possible to treat productivity as an objective variable if evaluators use a single, standardized instrument that reduces the prospect for subjective rankings. For example, the instrument could contain objective and quantitative measures, answering questions such as, *How many units did the employee produce in a 15-minute segment?* and *How many units were defective and had to be rejected?*

Using Specific Variables

Various quantifiable measures can be used as dependent variables to evaluate a worksite health promotion program. The general principles of choosing variables are covered in chapter 5; in this chapter, we are discussing unique points about using specific variables.

Participation As a Dependent Variable

Participation is probably the most common dependent variable used in organizational health promotion settings. Despite this distinction, participation is not necessarily a valid indicator of an intervention's impact. Its major limitation is that it only reflects the number or percentage of people attending or participating in a particular intervention. Thus, it does not signify their level of effort and progress toward achieving a goal. Participation is often defined quantitatively as

- number of total visits,
- number of total visits by age range or gender, or
- number of visits by employees versus dependents.

Despite its limitation, tracking participation can help program planners develop strategies to increase utilization levels, to identify natural cycles in program enrollment, and to make better scheduling decisions.

Participation can be measured by utilization, penetration, and adherence.

- **Utilization** is simply the number of individuals involved in program activities for a designated time frame. These counts can be used to identify peak participation periods, attendance cycles, and seasonal variation.

- **Penetration** is defined as utilization divided by the total population. The quotient of this procedure is a measure of how much the program has penetrated the total population, and it is called the **penetration rate**. The penetration rate is helpful when evaluating the success of targeting selected market segments—30-39-year-old women, for example.

- **Adherence** measures the regularity of participation and is often a good indicator of a program's impact. For example, adherence measures may include the number of employees with a minimum of two visits per week or the average number of visits per participating employee per month. Typically, at least half of the people who begin a new behavior do not continue with it long enough to reach their personal goal. Clearly, attaining high levels of adherence in an organizational setting is a challenge.

Absenteeism As a Dependent Variable

Absenteeism is one of the most ubiquitous dependent variables used in health promotion evaluations. Perhaps the most serious problem facing evaluators is defining a quantifiable measure of absenteeism. In the early 1960s, for example, researchers identified as many as 41 different absence measures. However, the Bureau of Labor Statistics (BLS) has developed three standard measures which are used by many organizations.

1. **Incidence rate** measures the number of absences per 100 employees during a given time period. Thus, the formula for establishing incidence rate is

$$\text{Incidence rate} = \frac{\text{number of workers absent}}{\text{total employees}} \times 100$$

For example, the incidence rate of an organization with 250 employees that has 15 workers absent in one (1) week would be figured like this:

$$\frac{15}{250} \times 100 = 6\%$$

Thus, for every 100 employees in this organization, six (6) were absent during the week.

2. **Absence rate** provides the percent of time lost due to absenteeism per 100 employees, so the formula for establishing absence rate is

$$\text{Absence rate} = \frac{\text{number of hours absent}}{\text{number of hours usually worked}} \times 100$$

For example, if 250 employees worked 40 hours per week and each of the 15 employees absent were off work for three (3) days (or 24 hours), the organization's absence rate would be figured like this:

$$\text{Absence rate} = \frac{15 \times 24 \text{ hours}}{250 \times 40 \text{ hours}} = \frac{360}{10,000} = 3.6\%$$

This indicates that 3.6% of the hours usually worked were lost due to employee absence.

3. **Severity rate** provides a measure of the average time that an absent employee loses during a given period. This variable can be treated as a percentage of usual hours worked. The formula for figuring severity rate would be

$$\text{Severity rate} = \frac{\text{average number of hours lost by absent employee}}{\text{average number of hours usually worked}} \times 100$$

For example, if three (3) employees were absent eight (8) hours, the severity rate would be

$$\text{Severity rate} = \frac{3 \times 8}{3 \times 40} \times 100 = \frac{24}{120} \times 100 = 20\%$$

Thus, 20% of the scheduled time was lost.

This variable can also be figured in absolute hours lost. In the case of the three (3) employees who were each absent for eight (8) hours, the absolute hours lost would, of course, be 24 hours.

There are many absence measurements that have been reported to be reliable in addition to the BLS measures that are described above. For example, common measures found in the literature include

- absence frequency (total number of times absent),
- absence severity (total number of one-day absences),
- attitudinal absence (frequency of one-day absences),
- medical absence (frequency of absences of three days or more),
- worst-day absences (difference between worst and best days absent), and
- blue Monday absence (number of employees absent on a Monday less those absent on a Friday).

Despite occasional problems in data quality, the relative ease in which absence data can be collected is probably the major reason for the abundance of literature on absenteeism, especially in personnel and human resources. The most common issues are self-selection bias, inconsistent definitions of absenteeism, and not differentiating between scheduled (planned) and unscheduled (unplanned) absences. If one can avoid such flaws in the data collection process, however, one can uncover significant relationships that can help WHP personnel plan effective programs. For example, 14 of the 20 articles reviewed by the author reported favorable effects of exercise on absenteeism—generally one to two fewer absences per year.

If absenteeism is used as a dependent variable, it should be clearly defined and quantified to coincide with the organization's record-keeping system.

They Say Po-tay-to, We Say Po-tah-to

A midsized organization experienced a significant increase in absenteeism, yet no one seemed to know what was causing the upward trend. Senior management instructed all departments to initiate programs, incentives, and policies to reduce this growing problem. The departments responded by establishing several company-wide initiatives within six months. After all of the initiatives had been fully operational for at least six months, senior management asked all departmental managers to report their progress. Unfortunately, however, the departmental managers could not provide any meaningful feedback because absenteeism had not been clearly defined or quantified at the time of the initial directive from senior management. Moreover, a formalized record-keeping system at the departmental level had not been established. Consequently, managers' progress reports contained no data, only personal observations and perceptions such as *I think absenteeism has dropped in my department*. Essentially, the managers' feedback provided no information on whether the various interventions had actually made an impact on absenteeism.

In retrospect, this unfortunate outcome could have been avoided if

- the causes of absenteeism had originally been identified and quantified, and
- an absenteeism tracking system had been established at the departmental level.

For instance, the personnel department manager should have established clearly defined categories of absenteeism—for example, scheduled (maternity leave, service on jury duty) versus unscheduled (sick leave, on-the-job injury). Second, absences should have been recorded according to categories within departments to determine the most common reasons for all types of absences. Finally, decision makers should have established an integrated health data management system to record and transmit absenteeism data from departmental managers to a central database (to the personnel department, e.g.).

By clearly defining, categorizing, quantifying, and transmitting absenteeism data, an organization can incorporate absenteeism more easily as an objective dependent variable in their evaluation efforts.

Financial	5%
Predictive factor: The ratio of employer-employee cost-sharing may encourage employees to misuse/abuse health care system	
Demographic	**7%**
Predictive factors: • Gender • Age > 45 years	
Morbidity	**26%**
Predictive factors: • Severe health problem • Multiple health problems • Chronic health problem • Existing health problem • Past history of health problem	
Clinical/behavioral	**29%**
Predictive factors: • Tobacco use • High blood pressure • High serum cholesterol • Physical inactivity • Obesity • Poor diet	
Attitudes/perceptions	**33%**
Predictive factors: • Pessimistic attitude toward life • Bad mood • Stressful experiences every day • Low confidence in doing medical self-care • Strong perceived need for health care • Lack social support system • No respect for high cost of health care • High dependence on health care system	

Figure 2.1 Health care utilization predictors by relative degree of influence.

Health Care Utilization As a Dependent Variable

Health care utilization is a measure that reflects the volume of or demand for health care services. It is usually quantified by tracking the number of health care claims incurred by employees and dependents.

Since the mid-1970s, many organizations have established utilization control strategies such as cost-sharing in their quest to reduce rising health care utilization and cost trends. This approach is based on the premise that unhealthy people are more likely to get sick and need health care services than healthy people; therefore, avoiding sickness will lessen the need for health care utilization. However, the data from most organizations shows that decreasing the sickness (morbidity) rate doesn't necessarily lead to less health care utilization. The reason is that utilization reflects the mind-set of a person consisting of behavioral, social, cultural, and financial factors (see figure 2.1) Health care utilization research conducted by the author and two colleagues suggests that use of health care services by employees and dependents is driven by no fewer than 22 factors, as seen in figure 2.1.

Since illness (morbidity) may account for less than one-third of all health care usage, should evaluation planners bother to track it? Definitely. Some researchers have reported short-term benefits of health promotion activities on specific types of illnesses and utilization barometers. How to track health care utilization through the use of claims data analysis is discussed in the next chapter.

What's It Worth?

A midsized manufacturing company experienced a significant rise in health care utilization for four consecutive years and summoned its health management personnel to investigate the problem. Upon closer review of the claims data, they found that the five most common types of claims were (in order of ranking) colds, low back injuries, depression, breast cancer, and hypertension. Unfortunately, the organization had no formalized worksite health promotion interventions targeted toward any of these conditions. As part of the organization's

(continued)

new cost-containment initiative, decision makers chose to target the three most common types of claims with new worksite-based interventions: First, a medical self-care program—consisting of a book, small group consumer information sessions, and monthly newsletters—was designed and targeted toward the prevention and treatment of colds and other upper respiratory tract infections. Second, a low back health program consisting of daily prework stretching sessions and proper lifting videos was targeted toward low back injuries. Finally, a confidential, toll-free hotline was established for employees and dependents with depression and other mental health concerns. Employee participation in each of the three interventions was as follows: medical self-care program, 90%; low back program, 50%; mental health hotline, 20%.

At the six-month evaluation, cold claims had dropped 5% from the preceding six months; back claims had dropped 20%; depression claims were virtually unchanged. Although the low back program had fewer participants than the medical self-care program, it produced a greater impact on health care utilization. Why? Because of associated risk factors and their level of modifiability. For instance, many low back claims are due to highly modifiable risk factors such as poor lifting, weak abdominal muscles, and low back flexibility, all of which can be influenced through appropriate worksite interventions. In contrast, colds and other acute respiratory tract infections are more difficult to prevent, much less quickly affect, because of the following two reasons: First, they are due to lifestyle and environmental risk factors (viruses, in particular) and thus occur in a much higher percentage of workers; second, they occur in workers of all ages, who can easily transmit these infections at the worksite. It is clear then that although health care utilization can be a viable dependent variable in a program evaluation, it must generally be used in connection with other dependent variables to be of maximum use (such as cost per claim and condition modifiability).

Risk Factor Status As a Dependent Variable

In the early 1960s, researchers began to quantify the effect of risk factors such as smoking and hypertension on rates of premature illness, disability, and death. In the late 1970s, organizations such as Kimberly-Clark Corporation, Quaker Oats Company, and Ceridian Corporation began to explore the impact of health risk status on health care usage and costs. They found that people with multiple risk factors incur more health care visits and costs than lower risk individuals (see figure 2.2). During the 1990s, several worksite studies reported anecdotal evidence that suggested a positive relationship between risk factor reduction and reduced health care costs. One of the most notable research efforts was an epidemiological study conducted on thousands of Chrysler Corporation employees by Dee Edington, PhD, of the University of Michigan. His research on the relationship between risk factor level and health care costs found the following:

- Workers with multiple risk factors incurred increasing health care costs with time.
- Workers who moved from low-risk factor status to high-risk factor status incurred greater health care costs.
- Workers who migrated from a high-risk factor profile to a low-risk factor profile incurred fewer health care costs.

Substantial evidence suggests that several risk factors also have a direct impact on productivity. Perhaps the most researched area is exercise with particular emphasis on physical inactivity as a strong risk factor. Numerous studies conducted during the

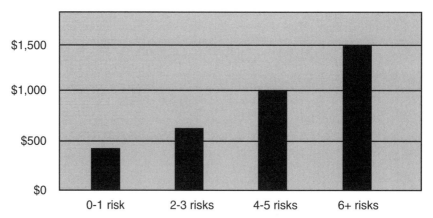

Figure 2.2 Approximate excess health care costs per risk factor.
Source: Health Management Associates database.

1980s showed that physically active employees obtain higher performance ratings than those in lower fitness categories; likewise, their injury rates and return-to-work times after an injury are better than less active workers. Moreover, studies of employee assistance programs (EAPs), stress management, and other mental health programs associated with health promotion demonstrate the positive effect of early intervention on both physical and mental productivity.

Risk factor status is influenced by

- lifestyle behavior,
- heredity/genetics,
- environmental exposures, and
- medical/health care delivery factors (see figure 2.3).

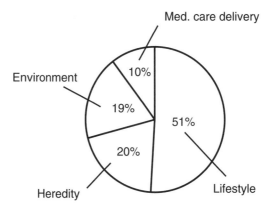

Figure 2.3 The approximate influence of specific influences on overall risk factor status.

Thus, if stakeholders are most interested in the bottom line, program planners should aim at risk factors known to have an economic effect, and program evaluation planners (usually the same people as the program planners) should aim to do three things:

1. Use risk factors as dependent variables when evaluating their respective programs.

2. Quantify the cost of the targeted risk factor either through an approach such as the *Proportionate Risk Factor Cost Appraisal* technique (see pages 73-77 in chapter 3) or by using a national norm to serve as the average cost per risk factor (see figure 2.4).

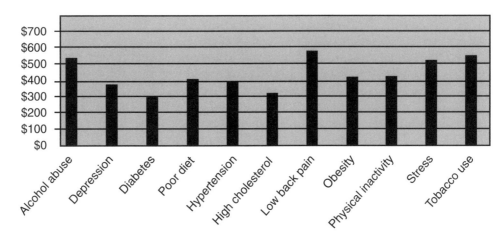

Figure 2.4 Median annual risk factor costs per employee per year.
Database sources: Crawford and Company, Health Management Associates, Health Evaluation and Research Organization, Milliman and Robertson, Inc., National Council on Compensation Insurance, and University of Michigan.

3. List the quantified risk factor as a baseline cost when the intervention begins, and make sure that a system is in place for careful tracking of any cost changes in this dependent variable. (Establishing a baseline is discussed in chapter 4 in connection with tools for financial analysis.)

How to use quantified risk factors as dependent variables in specific calculations is discussed in chapters 3 and 4.

Productivity As a Dependent Variable

Productivity is a component of performance, not a synonym for it. As our economy evolves from manufacturing-based to a service- and information-based marketplace, it is important to measure productivity in ways that reflect today's work styles. For the white-collar employees of departments such as research and development, logistics, strategic planning, and personnel, there are no widgets being produced, and no set number of sales calls to be made. In short, very few readily quantifiable and uniformly accepted measures of job performance exist for these types of positions.

In 1999, the American Productivity and Quality Center and The MEDSTAT Group collaborated on a national study of over 600,000 employees to identify and quantify the total cost of health and productivity-related issues to employers. They found that productivity losses cost employers an average of $9,992 per employee. This study's findings were strongly supported by a 1999 study conducted at Bank One Corporation by Wayne N. Burton, MD and Daniel J. Conti, PhD (see *Worker Productivity Index*).

Worker Productivity Index (WPI)

The **worker productivity index** (WPI) is a percentage that reflects the portion of scheduled work time an employee—or group of employees—is up to speed. The lower the number, the more time lost. We applied the index to more than 500 customer service workers at a major credit card company and calculated an average WPI of 89%. We then used it to show how health status affects output. We calculated the impact of specific diseases, chosen on the

(continued)

(continued)

basis of worker disability in the study year, health risks based on employee health risk appraisals (HRAs), and number of risks. In some cases, productivity was reduced by nearly a third.

Our findings lead to this conclusion: While it's crucial for employee health programs to target the sickest workers and the groups with the highest direct and indirect health costs, it's equally important to help the majority of employees at low risk stay that way. Despite the criticism that on-site gyms, healthy cafeteria food, and the like attract only those who would work out and eat well anyway, supporting the healthy is a vital—and considerably more profitable—way to keep health spending down and productivity up.

Exactly how is presenteeism measured? Not easily. Productivity studies are hampered by the difficulty of quantifying output, exacerbated by the shift from manufacturing and piecework to providing information and services. Matching productivity loss to individual risk factors is even harder, since it requires detailed employee health records. Enter First Card, a subsidiary of First Chicago NBD Corp., which merged with Banc One last year to form BANK ONE. A large number of the 3,000 employees at First Card's Elgin, Illinois, office provide telephone-based customer service. The company has a computer system that tracks time spent on various aspects of a call, time between calls to complete transactions and time logged off the system. All employees also have the opportunity to complete periodic HRAs. The results are stored in a database, along with everything from the worker's age, medical coverage, claims history and test results to participation in wellness programs and days lost to short-term disability and absenteeism, all encoded to ensure privacy. In our study, we included only workers who had completed HRAs. To arrive at the WPI, we set a productivity standard most employees would reach. We then measured the time lost to failure to maintain that standard on the job as well as time away from the job (the sum of scattered absences and STD [short term disability]). That added up to the total time lost, which we then divided by the number of weeks studied to get the average time lost each week. To compute the WPI, we divided that number by the scheduled work hours, then subtracted from 100%. A full-timer who averaged eight lost hours a week, for instance, would have a WPI of 80%. (8 hours divided by 40 equals 20 percent. Subtract that from 100%.)

In looking closely at the work/health connection, we found evidence of an interesting correlation: the fewer the health risks, the higher the productivity. Those with no more than one risk exceeded the group's average WPI by three points; those with three or more risks came in three points below average. We also made some discoveries: Among workers who had been on STD in the study year, those with digestive disease and mental health disorders had the lowest WPI scores. But the reasons were quite different. For example, those with digestive ailments were less likely to go on disability but more likely to suffer from presenteeism. The opposite was true for employees with mental health problems, who tended to perform well on the job but to lose lots of time to disability. Interestingly, smokers and couch potatoes had higher than average WPIs, but they have no reason to gloat. With an average age of 33, the workers studied are a bit too young to be showing the ill effects of smoking and a sedentary lifestyle. Diabetes was the risk factor most associated with the greatest productivity loss, followed by self-reported psychological distress and elevated body mass index. To employers with limited resources, studies like ours may seem like an impossible undertaking. But our next step, already under way, is to compare the workers' actual productivity with their estimates of output. Our aim is to create a simple formula many employers can use to yield similar findings.

Reprinted with permission from *Business & Health*, Vol. 17, No. 11, Medical Economics Company, Montvale, N.J.

When using productivity as a dependent variable, evaluators should address several issues:

1. They must **decide whether to measure qualitative-based or quantitative-based productivity outcomes**. For example, suppose an exercise-based stress management program has been successfully implemented in a white-collar setting such as an accounting, law, or financial consulting firm. Each of these settings would be appropriate for one or more of the following types of productivity measures:

- Qualitative Measures
  - Level of client satisfaction
  - Forecasting accuracy
  - Readability of educational literature
- Quantitative Measures
  - Number of new clients
  - Dollar value of recommended investments
  - Retention rate of clients

Likewise, productivity outcomes can also be qualitative or quantitative in blue-collar worksites such as construction, fast-food, and trucking. For example:

- Qualitative Measures
  - Building a home to exact specifications
  - Percentage of orders filled properly
  - Time to deliver goods safely
- Quantitative Measures
  - Number of homes built in one year
  - Number of orders filled in one hour
  - Truckloads delivered per week

2. They must **assess the feasibility of obtaining a valid measure of productivity at their worksite**. For example, evaluators will have to ask themselves, *Can we realistically and unobtrusively measure and quantify productivity?* Evaluators will have to consider issues of objectivity and validity here (pages 15-17 and 35-46). Common measurement techniques include the following examples:

- **Self-reported feedback.** Employees rate their perceived level of productivity on a survey.
- **External observation.** A supervisor rates an employee's performance.
- **Automated recording devices.** Computers record the number of units processed on an assembly line.
- **Internal tracking systems.** A personnel department database records every employee's sick leave absences.

3. They must **determine if there is a relationship between worker productivity and the specific intervention to be offered**. Evaluators need to ask, *What is the probability of the intervention boosting productivity?* and *What does the professional literature suggest?*

By addressing these issues, program planners and evaluators can be positioned to explore productivity as a useful dependent variable.

Working With Groups for Comparison

One of the most important decisions before conducting a good project effectiveness evaluation is identifying and selecting appropriate individuals and groups to evaluate. In many instances, an evaluation may be limited to participants because there is no comparable group of nonparticipants available. In some cases, logistical constraints prevail, and a shorter-than-usual intervention makes it impractical to recruit a control group. Regardless, the point is that an evaluation generally has more credibility when a control group or comparison group can be included.

Experimental and Control Groups

An evaluation is designed to determine what effects a program has on people. One way to do so is to select appropriate participant and nonparticipant sets of people. The group of individuals to be evaluated is known as the **experimental group** (the participants). A **control group** (the nonparticipants) should be used to make sure that the effects are caused by the program and not by some external factor. The control group should be as similar to the experimental group as possible, except that they do not receive the program intervention, or treatment, that is to be evaluated.

Without the use of a properly selected control group, the apparent effect of the program could actually be due to a variety of factors, such as differences in participants' educational background, environment, age, or experience. By using a control group, the likelihood is increased that the evaluation can determine whether results or outcomes are due to the program intervention or to other variables.

In an ideal situation, participants should be selected randomly then assigned randomly to one of two groups. Finally, it should be determined randomly which group would become the experimental group (participants) and which would become the control group (nonparticipants). Theoretically, this would evenly distribute the variables (such as age, gender, and race) among all groups and thus increase the credibility of the evaluation by controlling for extraneous factors. However, it is not always possible, or even ethical, to assign participants to a control group, especially if doing so would mean that they would be denied an essential program or service. For example, if a company has only one health promotion program designed for individuals with diabetes, denying some people with diabetes access to the program in order to form a control group would clearly be unethical.

One way to deal with this situation is to provide the control group with an alternative program or to offer them the regular program at a later time (if a delay is not potentially harmful). Another alternative is to compare two programs: Evaluators can offer an innovative program to some participants and continue the conventional program for others. This alternative enables evaluators to assess the effectiveness of the new program by comparing it with the old program.

A Lack of Control

A large manufacturing firm in the northeast had an aging workforce experience an annual claims increase of approximately 20%, including four coronary bypass claims that were responsible for 25% of the company's total claims costs. In response, decision makers decided to provide an on-site fitness facility, which they hoped would attract at-risk employees and thus significantly reduce their cardiovascular disease risk factors.

A survey was distributed to all employees to solicit their preferences for fitness center activities. Nearly 70% of the workforce responded. Program planners meticulously prepared programs and activities reflecting employees' interests. A one-group evaluation design was established with measurable outcomes tailored around health goals with particular emphasis on the most common risk factors, which were obesity, hypertension, and high cholesterol. Baseline risk factor status assessments were taken on 25% of the workforce who initially signed up for one or more of the programs. Follow-up, risk factor status assessments were taken at three months (December) and at six months (March). Both assessments showed 5% gains in participation and a significant reduction in each of the three targeted risk factors. Overall, the program was viewed as a major success with anticipation for an even greater impact in the future. Health promotion staff members appealed to the human resources director to hire another staff member to handle the projected demand for fitness center programs. Shortly thereafter, a new staff member was hired. Despite the initial growth in employee participation, however, evaluations conducted at 9 months and at 12 months showed virtually no growth in the number of new participants or reduction of risk factor levels.

At the company's annual meeting, the health promotion program director described each of the four evaluations and their results to senior managers. One manager wondered if the initial impact could have been due to the possibility that many participants were

- already taking personal risk-reduction actions and simply continued them while participating in fitness center programs,
- particularly motivated to exercise more in the cooler months (fall and winter) than in warmer weather, or
- motivated by New Year's resolutions to exercise more, eat better, and improve their health.

The health promotion program director admitted that these factors could indeed have influenced the risk-reduction actions more than the fitness center program alone and noted that, looking back, a control group (matched nonparticipants) should have been established to minimize the possible impact of outside influences on the evaluation results. By doing so, the evaluation would have provided decision makers with objective information to determine the real impact of the fitness center on each outcome goal.

Matching

What can you do when random assignment to a control group from the same pool from which the experimental group came is not possible? For example, suppose you have an experimental group composed of exercisers. You want to compare them with a control group of nonexercisers to see if physical activity influences absenteeism, yet you don't want to sensitize the nonexercisers to the fact that their absences will be tracked and compared with their peers' absences. Therefore, you must select an experimental group that will not be in close contact with the control group. In this case, a nonequivalent control group—also known as a **comparison group**—may be selected. Although it is not possible to have a completely equivalent group without random selection, it is important to form a group that is as similar as possible to the experimental group within the limitations of nonrandomization.

One of the most common ways to establish an acceptable level of similarity between experimental and comparison groups is **matching**. The first step in matching is to think of as many characteristics as possible that could affect the program results. Factors to consider may include participants' age, gender, education, health risk status, location within the company, socioeconomic status, and experience. The next step is to select a group that matches the experimental group with respect to each of these factors. This can be done on either a subject-to-subject or a group-to-group basis. Matching is particularly popular in ex post facto (after the fact) research in which evaluators need to construct a comparison group with similar characteristics to that of an already formed experimental group.

A variation of matching is also useful if you cannot use randomization to choose the experimental group. In this case, the best procedure is to use matching to come up with matched pairs, then assign each member to either the experimental or the comparison group through a random procedure, like tossing coins or using odd and even random numbers.

> **Computer Tip**
>
> In selecting variables to use in matching groups, consider reviewing case study abstracts of published articles that are available on the World Wide Web. Many professional associations provide free access to article abstracts that may provide information on co-relationships between specific variables. If you don't know the Web site address of a particular association, perform a search for a listing of relevant organizations.

REVIEW QUESTIONS: WORKING WITH GROUPS

1. What value can a control group provide in an evaluation?
2. What situations may keep evaluators from using random assignments?
3. How do you determine specific variables to use in matching comparison, control, and experimental groups?
4. What is the difference between a control group and a comparison group?

Working With Experimental and Non-Experimental Designs

If you wish to evaluate the effectiveness of a worksite health promotion intervention, the best way to do so is to plan the evaluation as you are planning the intervention. The clearest way of doing this is to select and apply a design to the intervention. In this context, a design is a structure for generating and collecting data on the effects of the intervention. Designs for program effectiveness evaluation can range from experimental to non-experimental. The text below presents evaluation designs which span this continuum. In the tables that illustrate each design, **O** refers to an observation or measurement, such as a survey, test, or interview. Measurement before the program begins is known as the pre-intervention, or pretest, and measurement after the completion of the program is known as the postintervention or post-test. **X** represents the program intervention. The relative positions of the two letters in the tables indicate when measurements are made in relation to when the program is provided. The tables also show which groups receive the program and when participants are randomly assigned to groups.

Experimental Designs

The most powerful type of design is the **experimental design** in which participants are randomly assigned to experimental and control groups. Experimental design offers the greatest control over extraneous factors that may influence the results. Potential disadvantages of the experimental designs are that they require a relatively large group of participants and that the intervention may be delayed for those in the control group. Moreover, experimental designs are time- and labor-intensive and may require informed consent from participants. The main challenge for evaluators is that such designs have to be applied under highly controlled conditions in which the behavioral circumstances are unusual or unnatural. For example, people who participate in a program that requires a change in behavior (e.g., exercise regularly, eat less fat, or reduce television watching) may experience stress and thus behave differently than they normally do. Therefore, evaluation outcomes may not be easily applicable to other organizational settings. In other words, although the rigorous procedures of an experimental design increase the validity of results, they may have limited feasibility and generalizability. Chapter 5, *Planning and Conducting Evaluations*, discusses how to apply these designs to specific projects.

Pretest–Post-Test and Post-Test Only Designs

The **pretest–post-test design** (figure 2.5) uses a pretest (O_1) to measure the participants before the program begins and a post-test at the conclusion of the program. Using a pretest not only provides a starting point for comparing measurements before and after the program, it also helps determine if the randomly assigned groups are indeed similar.

Pretest–post-test design

Experimental group	[R]	O_1			X		O_2
Control group	[R]						O_2

Post-test only design

Experimental group	[R]				X		O_1
Control group	[R]						O_1

Times series design

Experimental group	[R]	O_1	O_2	O_3	X			O_1
Control group	[R]	O_1	O_2	O_3	X	O_4	O_5	O_6

Staggered treatment design

Experimental group 1	[R]	X	O_1	O_2	O_3	O_4	O_5
Experimental group 2	[R]	O_1	X	O_2	O_3	O_4	
Experimental group 3	[R]	O_1	X	O_2	O_3		
Experimental group 4	[R]	X	O_1				

R = Random assignment
O = Observation/measurement
X = Program intervention

Figure 2.5 Experimental designs.

Some researchers believe the major advantage of the **post-test only design** over the pretest–post-test design is that the former avoids the effects attributable to testing the program participants. In this simple but powerful design, the differences between the post-test results (O_1) for the experimental and control groups can presumably be attributed to the intervention provided to the experimental group, assuming that the randomization procedure has achieved equality of the two groups before the participation of one group. Although randomization has become increasingly common as the chosen method of equalizing experimental and control groups, it is important to have an adequate number of people interested in the intervention to be randomly assigned to experimental and control groups. You may wish to consult a statistician or statistics book for sample size requirements after you have selected your dependent variables.

Time Series Design

A third pure experimental design is the **time series design**. This design can be used to examine differences in program effects over time. Random assignment to groups is necessary to establish control over factors influencing the validity of the results (see pages 35-40).

In a time series design, several measurements are taken over time before and after the program is implemented. This process helps identify other factors that may account for a change between the pretest and post-test measurements. It is especially appropriate for measuring delayed effects of a program. A time series design could be used in a weight-loss program to indicate the amount of weight lost over time and the ability to maintain a desired weight. This design could be used to evaluate and compare several types of programs, such as lecture, workshop, and self-study. Measurements could be collected from all groups at the same points in time, and programs could occur simultaneously.

Staggered Design

The **staggered design** is used to determine the effects of a program over time by including several measurements after the end of the program. It also indicates the effects of testing since not all groups in this design receive a pretest. The staggered treatment design can also be used in quasi-experimental and non-experimental designs but with the limitation of not using a control group.

Despite the unique features of a staggered design, some researchers feel that simultaneous designs (in which both groups receive pre- and post-tests at the same time) should be used in specific situations for two reasons. First, pretests and post-tests can be administered simultaneously for all groups, thus reducing the possibility of subtle changes in the administration of pretests and post-tests or other assessment methods. Second, with the staggered design, historical events may affect the groups differently. For example, if a television special on diabetes appeared on the air during the time period between pretest and post-tests, it would affect simultaneous groups equally, whereas it would affect staggered groups unequally. Randomization alone cannot protect the staggered design against exposure to different periods of history.

In spite of its disadvantages, there are times when a staggered treatment design is appropriate. For example, it should be used in the following circumstances:

- When an organization's resources (finances, personnel, facilities) are insufficient to offer several programs at the same time

- When the evaluator wants to see what effect an external event will have and thus needs groups whose experience will be the same, except for their exposure to an anticipated external event
- When the effects of testing need to be indicated since not all groups in this design receive a pretest

The staggered treatment design can also be used in quasi-experimental and non-experimental designs, though the limitations of not using a control group or comparison group will, of course, negatively affect the reliability of the results.

Quasi-Experimental Designs

Perhaps the most common type of evaluation design used in organizational health promotion settings is **quasi-experimental design** (figure 2.6). The prefix *quasi* means almost or nearly. Thus, a quasi-experimental design is similar to, but not as strong as, a true experimental design due to limitations in random selection. Although quasi-experimental designs can generate supportive evidence of a program's effectiveness, they cannot control for all factors that affect the validity of the results. There is no random assignment to the groups, and comparisons are made on experimental and comparison groups. Quasi-experimental design, using neither a comparison nor a control group, has little control over the factors affecting the validity of the results.

Quasi-Experimental Pretest–Post-Test Design

The **quasi-experimental pretest–post-test design** is often used when a control group cannot be formed by random assignment. In such a case, a comparison group (a nonequivalent control group) is identified, and both groups are measured before and after the program. For example, a program on physical fitness for employees could be evaluated by using a pre- and postprogram fitness test. Employees not receiving the program could serve as the comparison group. Similar pretest scores between the comparison and experimental groups would indicate the groups were equal at the beginning of the program. Without random assignment, of course, it would be impossible to be absolutely sure that other variables (e.g., offering financial incentives for exercising or distributing free exercise coupons) did not influence the results. However, if all other efforts are made to take possible extraneous factors into account, and if the numbers appear decisive, the evaluator can assure stakeholders that the results can be endorsed with a reasonable degree of confidence.

Pretest–post-test design						
Experimental group	O_1			X		O_2
Comparison group	O_1					O_2
Times series design						
Experimental group	O_1	O_2	O_3	X	O_4	O_5	O_6
Comparison group	O_1	O_2	O_3	X	O_4	O_5	O_6

O = Observation/measurement
X = Program intervention

Figure 2.6 Quasi-experimental designs.

Quasi-Experimental Time Series Design

The **quasi-experimental time series design** is structured like the experimental time series design, but it uses a nonequivalent comparison group. This design can be extended in the same way a staggered evaluation design is, adding more post-tests for the two groups, adding experimental groups to examine variations in the program, or both. The additional groups may be included with simultaneous alternative programs (if you have sufficient staff and facilities) or on a staggered basis. If several groups are added and receive interventions at different times, the design then becomes a quasi-experimental staggered treatment design.

Non-Experimental Designs

Non-experimental designs (figure 2.7) represent the third type of evaluation designs that are used in various organizational settings. Although it is the weakest of the three types, a non-experimental design is generally the only option when evaluators cannot assign participants to an experimental or control group, or there is no comparison group. Perhaps the most common non-experimental design is the **one group pretest–post-test design**. The major weakness of this simple design is that we cannot be sure that the results observed in O_2 could not have been caused by factors other than the program itself. For example, we have to ask if the results were influenced by

- extraneous events, such as a television program aired between O_1 and O_2 that has influenced the subjects' behavior;
- the growth and development of subjects that occurs with the mere passage of time between O_1 and O_2;
- the effect of O_1 on O_2 (that is, the experience with the test);
- changes in the measurement tools or procedures between O_1 and O_2; or
- interaction between the pretest and the program intervention. For example, the pretest itself may influence behavior by making participants aware of things they should or should not do.

To envision how external factors can threaten the validity of an evaluation, consider changes in the blood pressure of subjects who have completed a company-offered hypertension-control program. A decrease in the average blood pressure might mean that the program successfully motivated individuals to adopt healthy behaviors; however, it could also reveal the impact on people who read an article on hypertension in the company newspaper, who heard news of a stroke suffered by a well-known employee with hypertension, or who took advantage of the free blood pressure checks on company time. Having a comparison group, even if it is not a randomly selected or matched group, can minimize such threats to internal validity. As for the final example listed, the interaction between the pretest and the program intervention is a legitimate part of most health promotion programs. When we

Pretest–post-test design						
Experimental group	O_1			X		O_2
Times series design						
Experimental group	O_1	O_2	O_3	X	O_4	O_5	O_6

O = Observation/measurement
X = Program intervention

Figure 2.7 Non-experimental designs.

conduct pretest assessments for various baseline purposes, we should probably consider the direct and indirect effects of these tests as part of any program evaluation that is conducted with a non-experimental design.

In view of all the potential problems that non-experimental designs present, a single-group pretest–post-test design fails to offer a firm base for any conclusion about the effect of the health promotion program. It should be avoided if possible.

REVIEW QUESTIONS: EXPERIMENTAL AND NON-EXPERIMENTAL DESIGNS

1. What are the primary considerations in selecting an evaluation design?
2. What are the major strengths and weaknesses of various evaluation designs?
3. Discuss internal and external validity.
4. Why are experimental designs more powerful than other designs?
5. What is the purpose of a pretest in an evaluation design?
6. What type of design can be used to compare groups on several occasions before a program intervention begins?
7. Why are quasi-experimental designs more practical than experimental designs in many worksite settings?

Working With Data

We look at various issues involving data in later chapters, but in this one we discuss the differences among data, analysis, and information. We also discuss how to maximize your chances for obtaining valid data and how to design valid instruments for gathering qualitative data.

Computer Tip

Some organizations have such large medical claims data files that their insurers and third party administrators have to prepare them in comma delimited and other compressed formats. A powerful database management software program (i.e., SAS, SPSS, Filemaker, ACCESS) is often required to open, retrieve, and analyze such data formats. Before purchasing a database program, inquire about the size and format of the data to be analyzed to determine if you have the appropriate systems (hardware and software) to process it. Specifically, ask the software company about the hardware and software requirements for running the program, and be sure to upgrade as necessary before you try running the system on your machine.

Data, Analysis, and Information

Effective evaluation requires measurement, data, and analysis. **Measurement** is the process of assigning standardized quantitative terms to anything that can be described by such terms. In other words, measurement is the process of producing data, the quantitative basis of any evaluation effort. In their simplest form, **data** are numbers, percentages, and other quantitative units. Of course, data have to be analyzed in order to discover their significance. **Analysis** of data involves organizing them in the light of specific problems or questions, and it involves establishing relationships among the different groups of organized data. **Information** is defined as the significant conclusions that can be drawn from analyzed data. Without analysis, data may be meaningless or even misleading. Thus, measurement and analysis serve complementary roles in the evaluation process as illustrated in figure 2.8.

As the evaluator, then, it is your job to

1. analyze a situation in order to know what kind of data are needed;
2. request relevant data from outside sources, or set up an appropriate system to collect it in-house, or both;

3. gather the relevant data; and

4. analyze the data in order to produce useful information.

Such information is an indispensable resource for WHP planners. An example of how data are converted into information via the process of analysis is illustrated in figure 2.9. The details of this process are discussed at length in chapter 6.

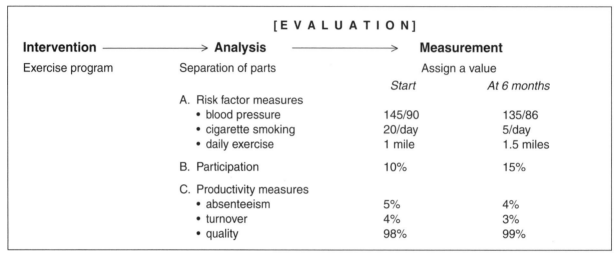

Figure 2.8 Role of measurement and analysis in evaluation.

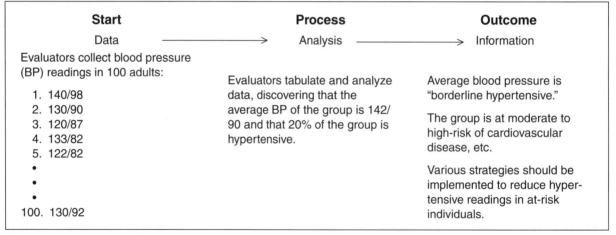

Figure 2.9 An example of data, analysis, and information.

Ignorance Isn't Bliss

Extracting information through analysis can make a difference in guiding an organization's worksite health promotion efforts. For instance, a large telecommunications company stored ten years of aggregate medical claims reports and, for various reasons, chose not to review the data. When the company's health management staff decided to plan its new employee health promotion program, the occupational health nurse recommended that various data sources—ranging from employees' health risk appraisals to medical claims reports—be reviewed to determine the most pressing employee needs and interests. Data reviews began,

(continued)

and a local consultant was hired to provide an independent review of medical claims reports covering the past decade. The three most common claims were (1) low back pain, (2) osteoarthritis, and (3) hypertension. All were strongly associated with an aging workforce, and all had ranked in the top five categories for the past five years. Yet there had been no on-site risk-reduction programs for any of these conditions available during this time frame. Based on this compelling evidence, a new, integrated risk-identification and management program was established for all employees with strong promotional efforts directed to those 40 years of age and above.

Analyses of the company's subsequent medical claims reports showed a drop in each of the targeted claim areas. By reviewing and extracting this valuable information, the organization was able to improve their employees' health status and contain a larger portion of its medical care tab.

Ensuring the Validity of Data

As is clear from our discussion of designs, how reliable evaluation results are—that is, their **validity**—is an important factor to consider in planning and executing WHP evaluations.

What Is Internal Validity?

The internal validity of a program evaluation is the degree to which we can demonstrate that the program caused any change in the dependent (outcome) variable. As noted above, many factors can threaten internal validity, either singly or in combination, making it difficult to determine if the outcome was due to the program or to some other cause.

Threats to Internal Validity

Some of the most common threats to validity in organizational settings are as follows:

- **Compensatory equalization** of treatments occurs when the program intervention is not available to the control group, and there is an unwillingness to tolerate the inequality. For instance, the control group may complain since they are not able to participate.

- **Compensatory rivalry** is when the control group is seen as the underdog and is motivated to work harder.

- **Diffusion, or imitation of treatments,** results when participants in the control group interact and learn from the experimental group. For example, workers randomly assigned to an ergonomics program (experimental group) may discuss the program with employees who are not in the program (control group) and thus bias the results.

- **History** occurs when an event happens between the pretest and post-test and is not part of the health promotion program. An example of history as a threat to internal validity is having a national antismoking campaign coincide with a worksite smoking cessation program.

- **Instrumentation** occurs when there is a change of measurement between pretest and post-test. This change includes the method of, the instruments used for, or the objects of measurement.

- **Maturation,** like history, is a threat primarily to designs that depend on pretest–post-test comparisons. Unlike history, maturation involves changes taking place within the individuals being measured over time, rather than the extraneous (nonprogram) events or changes taking place in the environment. The threat of maturation is particularly present when participants in the program may show pretest-to-post-test differences due to growing older, wiser, or stronger. It is most dramatically a threat, therefore, to evaluations of programs for children and youth, in whom maturational changes are more rapid. But it also plagues longitudinal studies of change in adults, especially studies centered on life span transitions such as graduation, marriage, family formation, divorce, midlife crises, retirement, relocation, and widowhood.

• **Mortality** refers to participants dropping out of the program between the pretest and post-test. For example, if most of the participants who drop out of a weight-loss program are those with the least (or the most) weight to lose, the group composition is different at the post-test. Such differences cannot be attributed entirely to the intervention but rather must be understood as a process of selection. As such, the loss of people from either experimental or control groups threatens internal validity.

• **Resentful demoralization of respondents** occurs when respondents receive less desirable treatments when compared with other groups and the resentment affects the outcome. For example, an evaluation to compare smoking cessation programs may assign one group (control) to the regular smoking cessation program and assign another group (experimental) to the regular program plus a financial incentive. If the participants in the control group become aware that the other group is receiving money that they are not being offered, they may resent the omission, and this may be reflected in their smoking behavior and attitude toward the regular program.

• **Statistical regression** occurs when groups have been selected on the basis of their extreme scores (which are not necessarily accurate). Consequently, any difference in the degree of shift from a pretest to a post-test between the two groups may actually be due to regression (a group's tendency to return—that is, regress—to their typical level of performance) rather than to the effect of the intervention. This threat is a particular danger in the pretest–post-test comparison group design.

• **Selection** reflects differences in the experimental and comparison groups, generally due to lack of randomization. Selection, then, is a threat to internal validity whenever the experimental and control or comparison groups are not identical. Any differences between the groups may account for their final differences on the dependent variables so that results could not be attributed solely to the intervention. Selection can also interact with other threats to validity, such as history, maturation, or instrumentation, which may appear to be program effects.

• **Interaction between selection and maturation** is another particular danger of a pretest–post-test comparison group design. For example, the groups may represent naturally assembled groups such as departments, as similar as availability permits yet not so similar that evaluators can dispense with the pretest. If the selection of groups results in distinctive differences in knowledge, skill, attitudes, or some other maturation-related attribute between the two parties, one group is inherently more likely to outperform the other on the basis on their pre-intervention maturation, not on the basis of the intervention. If, for example, the experimental group consists of exceptionally talented employees such as engineers or scientists, and it is compared with any readily available group with less talent or knowledge, interaction between selection and maturation is likely to occur.

• **Regression** occurs when groups have been selected on the basis of their extreme scores or performance. For example, suppose employees who may have joined the on-site fitness center because of a New Year's resolution are compared with a group of long-time fitness center participants. At the beginning of the evaluation time frame, the new members may have been as highly motivated to exercise as the long-time exercisers. However, enthusiasm typically wanes in new exercisers after several weeks, and thus, they return (regress) back to their nonparticipatory lifestyle. In such situations, the dropouts are no longer truly comparable to the long-term exercisers.

• **Testing** occurs when participants become familiar with the test format due to repeated testing. Using a different form of the same test for pretest and post-test comparisons will help minimize this effect.

• **Invalid instrumentation** occurs when instruments such as questionnaires or health risk appraisals are invalid; that is, they do not measure what they are supposed to measure. Exercise physiologists use the Balke or Bruce exercise stress test protocol to assess a person's cardiovascular fitness because both protocols are sensitive enough to accurately detect specific physiological indicators—such as heart rate, blood pressure, and so on—during a stress test session. If evaluators use a poorly designed protocol or one that is not appropriate for what they are trying to measure, they will not obtain accurate information.

Ruling Out Threats to Internal Validity

The major way in which threats to the internal validity of program evaluations can be controlled is through randomization. By random selection of participants, random assignment to groups, and random assignment of types of treatment (or no treatment) to groups, any differences between pretest and post-test can generally be interpreted as a result of the program. Of course, when random assignment to groups is not possible and quasi-experimental designs are used, the evaluator must make all threats to internal validity explicit and then take steps to minimize their influence. History and instrumentation are the two most common internal threats to the validity of a study using a quasi-experimental time series design.

• **History.** The longer the time between the pretest and post-test, the more likely it is that participants and nonparticipants will be exposed to personal and environmental forces that may have a greater influence than the intervention. Ideally, you should administer the post-test as soon as the intervention ends or as soon as enough time has lapsed from the beginning of the intervention for the program to have made an impact on the dependent variable. Perhaps best included under history—although in some sense akin to maturation—would be cycles such as the workweek, pay periods, vacations, special events, and the like. Thus, you should schedule measurements so that the cycles always have the same chronological relationship to the measurements or else far enough apart to include such cycles in their entirety.

• **Instrumentation.** The time series design is used frequently to measure the effects of a change in programming or policy. Bearing this in mind, evaluators would be wise to avoid changing their measuring instruments or techniques at the time of any programming or policy change. Suppose, for example, that an organization expanded its medical self-care program to include a telephone hotline to guide employees and dependents in their health care decisions. Before the expansion, evaluators measured health care utilization of employees and dependents to determine which group incurred the greater number of medical claims. Their baseline measurements were, of course, based on this measurement method. However, shortly after the program expansion occurred, a new benefits director was hired and instructed the staff to measure the impact of the program on medical care expenses (rather than claims) and to count only those expenses associated with employees. Even though the evaluation had been set up with randomly selected experimental and control groups, this change in what was being measured made it impossible to accurately determine the impact of the expanded program on health care utilization. The measurement parameters for health care utilization became different from those used to establish the baseline. This conflict could have been avoided if the new benefits director had understood that changing what was measured caused any results from the study to be useless because of the instrumentation threat to validity.

The pretest–post-test comparison group design has two potential threats to internal validity that reside between selection and maturation. These threats—regression and interaction—must be addressed because the design includes two groups that do not necessarily have pre-intervention equivalence. To counter these potential threats, you should consider using pretest differences in selecting, if necessary, another comparison group that more closely resembles the experimental group on key attributes.

What Is External Validity?

The other type of validity that should be considered when deciding how to evaluate program effectiveness is external validity. **External validity** is also known as generalizability and is the extent to which the program intervention can be expected to produce similar effects in other populations. Generalizability is a particular concern when a program intervention is tailored to a specified population. For example, suppose you offered a group of assembly-line workers a smoking cessation program consisting exclusively of a nicotine replacement device (nicotine gum or patch) that produced a 33% success rate. Could you reasonably expect a similar success rate using the same approach with clerical personnel? Or assembly-line workers at another worksite? The more a program intervention is customized to a particular population, the greater the threat to external validity and the less likely it is that the program can be generalized to another group.

Back to the Drawing Board

A large manufacturing company developed a low back injury prevention program for its management personnel, which made up 10% of the workforce. The program consisted of

- weekly e-mail messages on the importance of a healthy back;
- monthly biomechanical assessments conducted by the occupational health nurse; and
- a daily, five-minute, prework stretching routine performed on company time.

The program generated widescale participation and produced impressive reductions in low back injuries and associated costs within six months of its inception. The corporate medical director reported the impressive findings to the president and predicted that even greater results would occur if the program were offered to the entire workforce. Upon hearing this lofty projection, the president decided to solicit independent feedback from an external consultant to determine the probability that the prediction was accurate.

The consultant explained that the initial findings could not be generalized to the entire workforce because the initial program was too customized around the work patterns and resources of a small percentage of the entire workforce. For example, the original program did not account for the following facts:

- Most employees did not have access to on-the-job e-mail announcements.
- Offering biomechanical assessments to all employees would be time prohibitive for the company's sole nurse.
- Assembly-line operations could be seriously jeopardized if employees left their work stations for varying periods of time to be assessed.

(continued)

The consultant indicated, however, that had the initial program been designed with enough latitude to meet the needs of all employees, the conclusions could have been generalizable to the entire company. To achieve this level of generalization, the program needed to do the following:

- Provide daily informational messages at strategically positioned locations accessible by all employees, such as the company entrance, time clock, cafeteria, and restrooms.
- Establish a schedule in which all employees could receive a personal biomechanical assessment every six months.
- Design a rotating, prework stretching schedule for all employees to complete in the first 15 minutes of their own shifts, thus avoiding assembly-line downtime.

The consultant suggested that the company run another pilot study on a different group using the features suggested above. By doing so, valid conclusions could be drawn about subsequent programs and their participants.

Threats to External Validity

As with internal validity, several factors can threaten external validity. These factors are sometimes known as reactive effects since they cause people to react in a certain way.

- The **expectancy effect** occurs when attitudes projected onto individuals cause them to act in a certain way. For example, in a weight management program, the instructor may feel that a certain person will not benefit from the intervention; projecting this attitude may cause the person to behave in self-defeating ways.

- The **Hawthorne effect** is named after an experiment in industrial hygiene at the Hawthorne Electrical plant in Chicago. Workers seemed to increase their productivity when the lighting was increased, and they also increased their productivity when the lighting was lowered. The evaluators concluded that the workers were responding favorably to the attention being paid to them. This interpretation has been debated, but the possibility of making your results unrepresentative by paying too much attention to your subjects remains a threat to external validity.

- The **placebo effect** happens when people improve because they believe in the intervention. This effect is so common in medical research that control groups are routinely given a placebo treatment to equalize their tendency to respond favorably due to the belief that any treatment given by the doctor will improve their condition. In organizational health settings, the placebo effect can occur even without medicines or surgical procedures if program staff members wield enough influence to change attitude or behavior apart from the educational effect. When the believer is the educator, the effect is called the Pygmalion effect.

- The **Pygmalion effect** is named after the mythical Greek king Pygmalion, who sculpted a stone woman so ideal that he fell in love with his work. Venus, taking pity on him, turned his stone beauty into a real woman. Thus, the Pygmalion effect is the belief that if one expects something to happen strongly enough, it can and will happen. Both positive and negative applications of this effect have been shown.

- The **sentinel effect** occurs when a person, upon seeing or suspecting others are watching him, acts in accordance with their expectations. For example, suppose a company is experiencing financial hardships because of excessive overhead and low productivity. Management sends a memorandum to all employees informing them that supervisors will be monitoring productivity on an hourly basis via visual observations and computer checks. Under these circumstances, employees sense the need to be more productive and improve their output.

- The **social desirability effect** is when the subjects, wanting to please or impress the evaluator, give answers or demonstrate behavior that they think is expected of them. This effect is especially common in situations where the evaluator is also the teacher, doctor, employer, or other person controlling rewards for the subjects. For example, an employee tells his substance abuse counselor that he has significantly decreased his alcohol consumption, when in fact he has not.

- **Inappropriate sampling** occurs when evaluators inadvertently select a sample of people who do not match the characteristics of the experimental group.

External validity can also be jeopardized by interactions between two or more factors. Examples include the following:

- **Selection and treatment.** A program requiring a large time commitment may not be generalizable to individuals who do not have much free time.

- **Setting and treatment.** Evaluation results from a program conducted on campus may not be generalizable to the worksite.

- **History and treatment.** Results from a program conducted on a historically significant day may not be generalizable to other days. For example, many worksites provide smoking cessation programs, activities, and incentives around the Great American Smokeout (the third Thursday in November). Many smokers successfully quit for the day but return to smoking soon after the program or incentives end.

Reducing Threats to External Validity

How can you reduce the preceding threats to external validity? Conducting the program several times in a variety of settings with a variety of participants can reduce many of these threats. Threats to external validity can also be counteracted by making a greater effort to treat all subjects identically. In a blind study, the participants do not know which group is the control group and which is the experimental group. In a double-blind study, neither the participants nor the program planners know the type of group the participants are in. In a triple-blind study, this information is not available to the participants, planners, or evaluators. Overall, a blind study is more feasible in an organizational setting than a double- or triple-blind study.

It is important to select an evaluation design that provides both internal and external validity. This may be difficult since lowering the threat to one type of validity may actually increase the threat to the other. For example, tighter evaluation controls that characterize all true experimental and some quasi-experimental designs make it more difficult to generalize the results to other situations. One must walk the narrow line of exerting enough control over the evaluation to allow interpretation of the findings while allowing sufficient flexibility in the program to permit the results to be generalized to similar settings.

Designing Instruments for Gathering Qualitative Data

Worksite health management personnel use various tools to measure employees' health status, knowledge, attitudes, interests, needs, and behaviors. Some common instruments include health risk appraisals, questionnaires, surveys, and direct observations. Because each of these tools plays an important role in providing decision makers with key information, it is crucial that they be valid; that is, they must measure what they are supposed to measure. Using a valid instrument increases the chances that planners will rule out incorrect explanations for the results.

If possible, evaluators should use standardized instruments that have already been validated by the vendor or manufacturer. This requires obtaining permission from the copyright owner if the document is not in the public domain. The advantages of using measuring instruments that have been developed by experts include increased credibility, lower cost, less planning time, and more assurance of validity and reliability. Of course, the main disadvantage—one that prevents the use of standardized questionnaires in many cases—is that not all the items used to measure a particular aspect of a person's health status may be relevant or appropriate to use in all workplace settings. If you are considering using a standardized instrument, ask vendors what level of validity has been established for a particular instrument. A value of .70 or above is generally an acceptable level of validity (1.0 is maximum).

If you are designing your own instrument for gathering quantitative data, you must consider two major types of validity: content validity and criterion-based validity.

- **Content validity** requires that the instrument include items from each primary area of desired information. A review of the professional literature is a good first step toward establishing content validity since current information about the topic must be used to develop the instrument. For example, when planning to measure the cardiovascular disease risk of a workforce, you can conduct a review of the professional literature or consult a jury of experts in the area of cardiovascular disease to ensure that every factor currently understood to increase the risk of cardiovascular disease is listed on the assessment tool you are developing.

- **Criterion-based validity** is determined by established criteria and looks at the relationship between two aspects of the same phenomenon. **Concurrent validity** is of concern when the two measurements are focused on the relationship between two current factors, such as scores on a knowledge test about cardiovascular disease and current exercise habits. If the measurement used will be correlated with a future measurement of the same phenomenon, such as using health care costs to predict future health care utilization, the criterion-based validity is known as **predictive validity**. The level of predictive validity or invalidity will not be known until multiple evaluations using the selected instrument have been completed. Once that has happened, evaluators can use these findings to determine if the instrument is acceptable or if other variables need to be integrated for future evaluations.

Validity in Self-Report Instruments

Bias is a major threat to the validity of an instrument. Bias is the difference between the response obtained and what is actually true. Although bias is a potential threat in virtually all measurement tools, it is particularly strong in self-report instruments. Thus, the presentation, wording, and sequence of questions in self-report questionnaires and interviews can be critical in gaining the necessary information. For instance, the questionnaire or interview should begin with a preface explaining the purpose of the technique and why the responses are important. The actual questions used in these tools should be clear and should not imply what answer the evaluator is hoping to hear. It is important to avoid questions with a specific direction (*How much have you enjoyed the fitness center?*) that would guide the respondent's answer. In addition, two-part (double-barreled) questions should be avoided (*Do you exercise and have a healthy diet?*). Another problem with question design occurs when the question assumes knowledge that people may not have or includes terms they may not understand (*How many health plan dividend dollars did you earn by participating in the medical self-care program?*). Unstructured or open-ended questions—such as essay, short-answer questions, journals, or logs—may be used to gain descriptive information about a person's health status or behavior, but they are generally not used to solicit qualitative data because they are often difficult to summarize or code for analysis.

If you plan to use self-report measurement tools, evaluation experts recommend that you do the following:

1. Select measures that clearly reflect program goals.
2. Select measurement instruments that have been designed to minimize biased responses and have been validated by qualified authorities.
3. Conduct a pilot study first with a portion of the target population.
4. Anticipate and correct possible sources of invalidity and unreliability in the measurement tool.
5. Use quality control procedures to detect possible cases of misinterpretation and miscoding. For example, review all evaluation results at specific intervals to detect any abnormal findings.
6. Use multiple types of measurement instruments with the same group, if possible, to minimize pretest bias.
7. Conduct two or more measurements to determine if any changes have occurred.
8. Use experimental and control groups with random assignment, when possible, to control for biases.

Validity in Direct Observation

Direct observation is often used by evaluators to obtain information on the behavior of individuals to determine their risk status. For example, evaluators might observe employees in the cafeteria to gain information about actual food choices and consumption. This method can be time-consuming, yet it is generally more accurate than self-report. Nonetheless, just the physical presence of an observer may alter the behavior of the people being observed. For instance, having someone observe lifting techniques may cause employees to be more conscientious and demonstrate proper lifting procedures due to the Hawthorne effect or sentinel effect. Thus, observers must be as inconspicuous and unobtrusive as possible in order to minimize measurement bias. Direct observation cannot eliminate subjectivity altogether, which can reduce the level of validity in the measurement process. One way to minimize the impact of subjectivity bias in a measurement is to have measurements taken by multiple observers, using the same instrument, and then compare their observations. If the observers' measurements differ substantially, it will be necessary to try different instruments until one is found that yields greater consistency among the observers. A second way to minimize subjectivity bias is to administer multiple types of measurement instruments to a target population, tabulate the scores into a single group mean (average) or median (50th percentile), and use this middle-of-the-road measure as the score. This technique will prevent low-end and high-end scores from inflating the representative norm of a population.

Validity is the cornerstone for establishing a good measurement tool that will yield the accurate information needed to make good baseline, progress, and outcome decisions. By incorporating the procedures outlined in this section, you can increase the validity of your measurement instruments.

Analyzing Qualitative Data

Once you obtain qualitative data from a survey or questionnaire, how do you analyze it? That depends on the format and type of data obtained as well as the types of

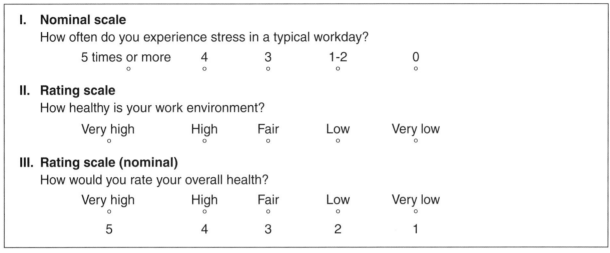

Figure 2.10 Sample HRA formats.

analytical resources available. Ideally, these factors should be considered before specific instruments are used because data formats can vary significantly from instrument to instrument. Take health risk appraisals (HRAs), for example. There are over 50 different HRAs in today's marketplace, ranging from single-page, self-scored formats to comprehensive 50-plus page, computer analyzed formats. Common content items found on some HRAs may appear in one or more of the formats shown in figure 2.10.

Note that the first and third scales have a numerical value attached to each option, making it relatively easy to ascertain how a respondent quantitatively views his situation. However, the second scale does not have a numerical value attached to each option. Therefore, if on-site evaluators wanted a quantitative index of a respondent's status, they would have to manually affix numerical values to each response option before they (or off-site evaluators) analyze each instrument. Ideally, it pays to consider these formatting issues before selecting a particular instrument. Otherwise, decision makers may end up selecting a vaguely developed instrument that requires additional work by on-site or off-site evaluators, which can lead to additional costs.

A central issue facing any worksite is deciding on whether in-house personnel have the capabilities to analyze specific instruments. Worksites who prefer to keep these analyses in-house may develop their own instruments or select commercial formats that can be scanned and analyzed by in-house personnel. Perhaps the best example of this arrangement is the growing number of companies who have purchased or leased scanning software and hardware from commercial vendors that permit them to do the bulk of HRA data entry and analysis in-house. Still other organizations prefer to pay commercial vendors to handle these tasks.

As more organizations opt to have greater in-house control over the selection of their instruments and associated analyses, they often find that developing a new instrument can be quite challenging. When developing a new instrument, it is important that the tool be valid, reliable, and prepared for easy analysis. For example, note that questions 2-10 on the Worksite Environment Survey in figure 2.11 are arranged in order of value (5-4-3-2-1) from left to right. The numerical values provide some measure of quantification to be assigned each item.

Computer Tip

When purchasing a scanner, first research scanning software to determine the variety and price options. Then, based on software options available, select a software package and prepare the scannable document so that it can be read by the software. Finally, select the appropriate hardware (computer) that is compatible with the software package selected. By using the software-first approach, you can avoid selecting hardware that may not be compatible with the scanning software.

Worksite Environment Survey

Instructions: Please answer each question by filling in the appropriate bubble (°).

1. I work primarily (select one)   °Indoors   °Outdoors

2. My employer's commitment toward a healthy worksite is:

Very high	High	Moderate	Low	Very low
°	°	°	°	°
5	4	3	2	1

3. The air quality at my worksite is:

Very high	High	Moderate	Low	Very low
°	°	°	°	°
5	4	3	2	1

4. The temperature at my worksite is:

Very good	Good	Moderate	Poor	Very poor
°	°	°	°	°
5	4	3	2	1

5. The quality of lighting at my worksite is:

Very good	Good	Moderate	Poor	Very poor
°	°	°	°	°
5	4	3	2	1

6. The level of security and personal safety I feel at my worksite is:

Very good	Good	Moderate	Poor	Very poor
°	°	°	°	°
5	4	3	2	1

7. The level of safety awareness and accident prevention at my worksite is:

Very good	Good	Moderate	Poor	Very poor
°	°	°	°	°
5	4	3	2	1

8. My employer provides me with safety information and resources:

Very often	Often	Sometimes	Rarely	Never
°	°	°	°	°
5	4	3	2	1

9. My co-workers practice safety at the worksite:

Very often	Often	Sometimes	Rarely	Never
°	°	°	°	°
5	4	3	2	1

10. My employer recognizes employees for safe work practices:

Very often	Often	Sometimes	Rarely	Never
°	°	°	°	°
5	4	3	2	1

Figure 2.11   A worksite environment survey that is valid, reliable, and prepared for easy analysis.

With the same numerical values arranged in a consistent direction (left to right), it is easy for each response to be manually or electronically recorded, analyzed, and tabulated. Nominal formats can be analyzed using simple row-by-row and tabulation procedures. First, construct a sample sheet for recording responses such as the one shown in figure 2.12.

Second, suppose 50 employees complete a survey with some variability from item to item. List the number of responses per item corresponding to each row and column, then multiply the number of responses by the row value (5-4-3-2-1) in order to calculate the total (211), divide the total by the number of respondents (50) and compute the average (4.22). Figure 2.13 provides an abbreviated example.

The preceding approach is a simple yet effective way to manually calculate the value of each item when doing an in-house analysis.

	#	#	#	#	#
1.	N/A				
2.	___	___	___	___	___
3.	___	___	___	___	___
4.	___	___	___	___	___
5.	___	___	___	___	___
6.	___	___	___	___	___
7.	___	___	___	___	___
8.	___	___	___	___	___
9.	___	___	___	___	___
10.	___	___	___	___	___

Figure 2.12 Sample tabulation sheet.

	# (5)	# (4)	# (3)	# (2)	# (1)	Row total	Avg.
1.	N/A	N/A	N/A	N/A	N/A		
2.	20	25	2	2	1		
3.	15	15	10	5	5		
4.	17	13	10	8	2		
5.	15	13	12	7	3		
6.	18	12	16	2	2		
7.	14	8	10	10	8		
8.	15	14	12	5	4		
9.	12	12	10	9	7		
10.	19	18	5	6	2		

Figure 2.13 Sample tabulation sheet calculations.

REVIEW QUESTIONS: WORKING WITH DATA

1. Why are data meaningless without analysis?
2. What are several potential threats to the internal validity of an evaluation?
3. What factors can jeopardize external validity?
4. What factors should be considered in selecting a standardized measurement instrument?
5. How do you analyze qualitative data vs. quantitative data?

CHAPTER REVIEW

Summary

Early in the program planning phase, careful consideration should be given to the evaluation of that program. This will help to ensure that the evaluation is focused on the goals and objectives of the program and will allow evaluators to assess the availability of essential resources. If an evaluation is to be conducted by external personnel, program planners should consult with them early to match the scope and specificity of the evaluation with outcome variables that coincide with the program's goals. Such collaboration makes it more likely that an appropriate evaluation design can be selected to incorporate experimental, control, or comparison groups. Issues such as randomization and matching should also be considered in determining if multiple groups will be included in an evaluation. Then, various data analysis techniques can be considered to convert data into strategic information. Chapters 3 and 4 present an overview of non-econometric and econometric evaluation frameworks.

What Would You Do?

1. You have recently been promoted and will assume more responsibility for evaluating the effectiveness of your company's employee health promotion program. Previous evaluations centered primarily on participation rates measured at semi-annual intervals. Your supervisor has asked you to expand the scope of your evaluation efforts to include a control group of nonparticipants. Naturally, you are concerned about selecting a comparable group of nonparticipants to ensure an apples-to-apples comparison. In doing so, you plan to apply a matching procedure throughout the entire organization to develop a comparable group of nonparticipants. Your rationale is that 60% of current participants represent 90% of all departments. The remaining 40% of participants are management personnel. Also, you strongly feel that quarterly evaluation intervals (every three months) would be better than semiannual evaluations. Your supervisor suggests that any matching procedures to be conducted should be restricted to management personnel because, in her view, they are administratively easier to match through the company's database and representative of most participants. To persuade her to adopt your preferences on both the comparison group and the evaluation intervals, what would you say?

2. You have recently been assigned to develop a proposal for evaluating your WHP program. Upon serious review of the current programs, you decide that the evaluation framework should consist of, in part, three outcome variables: employees' cardiovascular risk factor status, cardiovascular-based medical care claims, and absenteeism tied to cardiovascular disease risk factors. You design a one-group, pretest–post-test

design that will include a baseline measurement followed by a post-test evaluation in four months. Despite your good intentions to develop a sound evaluation plan, your colleagues ask the following questions when they see your proposal:

1. How will cardiovascular risk factor-based absences be distinguished from other causes of absenteeism?

2. Isn't four months too short a time frame to see tangible changes in the outcome variables?

3. By using a non-experimental design, how will we know if any changes are really due to the WHP program rather than to extraneous factors?

4. Wouldn't it be better to hire an outside consultant to conduct an evaluation that will be viewed as more objective by senior management?

You respect your colleagues deeply and must, therefore, consider their questions carefully. What will your answers be?

PART II
Instruments of Analysis

3

Project Effectiveness Analysis

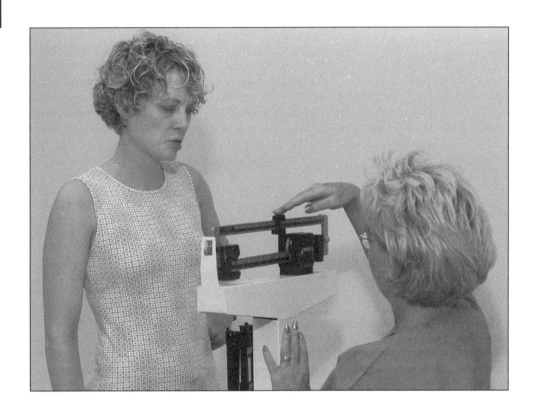

After reading this chapter and answering the questions at the end, you should be able to do the following:

- Distinguish between a claims data analysis (CDA) and a risk factor cost appraisal.

- Identify how a CDA can be used by various health management personnel.

- List at least three ways of classifying health claims data.

- List several requirements for doing an in-house CDA.

- Explain the step-by-step procedures used in each of the major phases for doing a CDA.

- Explain the primary purpose for doing a risk factor cost appraisal.

- Explain step-by-step procedures for doing a risk factor cost appraisal.

There are two broad categories of standard tools for data analysis: non-econometric and econometric. **Non-econometric** tools comprise primarily straightforward numerical data—for example, number of participants, prevalence rates, percentage comparisons. The data sources for all these types of analysis are health care claims. Thus, both of the non-econometric tools discussed in this chapter can be considered to be claims data analysis. In spite of that, it is accepted terminology in the field to call the more general procedure discussed first simply *claims data analysis* while the second is known as *risk factor cost appraisal*.

In contrast, cost-effectiveness analysis, break-even analysis, benefit-cost analysis, and forecasting are known as **econometric** tools because they rely on more complex types of data or statistical formulas to explore relationships between and among certain variables. Whereas many researchers use the term *economic* to refer to these tools, the author prefers the term *econometric* because it denotes the application of statistical methods to the study of economic data and problems.

Analyzing qualitative data comprises a third category of data analysis. Although analyzing qualitative data does not involve standardized tools, it does require that careful procedures be followed to obtain valid results.

This chapter presents the non-econometric claims data analysis tools (claims data analysis and risk factor cost appraisal) and discusses the principles of analyzing qualitative data. Chapter 4 discusses the econometric tools for analysis, including forecasting, which, because it uses data from medical claims, could be considered a form of claims data analysis in spite of the fact that the accepted terminology does not reflect this.

Claims Data Analysis

As the issue of cost-justification has intensified at most worksites so has the demand that health promotion programs be carefully planned and intelligently targeted. Analyzing the data made available through tracking employee health care insurance claims is an important tool in the repertoire of the evaluator, providing valuable information for improved planning and targeting. In this chapter, we look first at what CDAs may be used for, then we explain how the data on claims are classified. Afterward, we look at how to decide whether to do a CDA in-house or to turn to outside resources. Finally, we go through the step-by-step phases of a CDA.

Applications of CDA

Health care **claims data analysis** (CDA) can be an effective tool for discovering what health promotion services are needed. For instance, an organization's claims data report might reveal the following:

- Low back injuries are rising.
- Ankle sprains among warehouse workers are doubling every six months.
- Complications associated with pregnancy are rising.
- The number of questionable emergency room visits is increasing.

These data would give the organization's health management personnel clear targets to address, leading to the development of such measures as follows:

- The fitness center manager could increase the availability of low back equipment and provide instruction on how to use it.
- The safety manager could conduct a thorough environmental assessment of the warehouse to determine possible reasons for the rise in ankle injuries.

- The occupational health nurse could establish a comprehensive prenatal health education program to reduce the potential for pregnancy-related complications.

- The health promotion specialist could design and implement a lunch-'n'-learn series on medical self-care to help employees distinguish a real emergency versus a nonemergency.

CDA can also be used in process, impact, and outcome-based evaluations. For example, an organization has detected a significant rise in the number of employees using various orthopedic specialists to treat their musculoskeletal ailments. The wide-scale use of specialists has resulted in significantly higher medical payments by the organization. Based on these disturbing results, the organization has decided to contract with a single orthopedic group who agreed to offer discounted fees for treating the organization's employees. In addition, the employer has agreed to pay 90% of employees' medical care versus only 50% at other orthopedic groups. By offering this single-provider, financial-incentive approach, the employer hopes to motivate the vast majority, if not all, of its employees to use the contracted provider of choice. How will they tell if this approach is working or not? By using CDA to do a periodic process evaluation. Through monitoring employees' musculoskeletal claim and charge data on, say, a quarterly basis, the employer can regularly track claims and thus determine if a high percentage of employees are using the contracted orthopedic facility.

CDA can also be a good tool to use in an impact evaluation. For instance, a quarterly process evaluation could be supplemented with semiannual data to see if the intermediate impact is better than, similar to, or worse than the earlier evaluation. Semiannual data often provide decision makers with a more accurate view of the success or failure of a program or activity than do shorter-term periodic reviews, enabling evaluators to revise or eliminate interventions with some confidence.

Finally, CDA is a good tool for an outcome evaluation, which includes one or more outcome goals for a particular intervention. For instance, assume an organization identified a substantial rise in emergency claims among its employees in the past year. The organization responded by developing a comprehensive medical self-care program consisting of employee self-care booklets, educational seminars conducted in weekly safety meetings, and financial incentives tied to actual claims data results. The primary goal of this program was to reduce the number of emergency claims filed by employees. Using semiannual and annual claims data reports as part of an outcome evaluation, the organization can determine if the number of emergency claims has dropped. Moreover, decision makers can use these comparative results to decide whether future medical self-care programs should continue the approach of the current program or need to be substantially changed.

Ways of Classifying Health Care Claim Data

Before requesting medical claims data from an insurer or third-party claim administrators (TPA), it's important to be familiar with the standard types of medical claims forms provided to employers. Many employer medical claims reports are formatted with one or more of the following classifications:

- **Major Diagnostic Category** (**MDC**). A broad category that reflects various medical conditions, illnesses, or disabilities usually related to a single body system, such as circulatory, respiratory, and so on.

- **International Classification of Disease** (**ICD**). A specific type of medical condition, illness, or disability within a specific MDC. For example, arthritis is an ICD within the MDC known as musculoskeletal.

Computer Tip

When researching different database software programs, check to see if a particular program allows you to easily create integrated data records to explore possible relationships. For example, does the program provide mechanisms for doing correlational analyses between multiple types of data—age and low back claims, gender and health care costs, job title and participation in certain programs? Give each vendor sample data and ask them to describe how their program would extract, import, and analyze the data to generate an outcome.

• **Diagnostic Related Group (DRG)**. A group of similar diagnostic conditions, illnesses, or disabilities usually related to a specific body system. For example, DRG #243 (backache) represents several types of back ailments, ranging from simple backache to back strain/sprain.

Most employers receive their claims data formatted by major diagnostic categories (MDCs). Depending on the formatting practices of an insurer or claims administrator, the scope of claims reports provided to an employer may range from 17 MDCs to as many as 25 different MDCs.

Major Diagnostic Categories

The U.S. Department of Health and Human Services and the Health Care Financing Administration originally conceived MDCs as a complete slate of categories for the medical and insurance communities. Thus, it is generally assumed that TPAs and insurers will include all of them in their corporate claims reports. However, depending on a TPA's or insurer's database setup, data tracking and reporting philosophy, and a number of other factors, TPAs and insurers may elect to

- use all of these MDCs,
- include only those that have one or more claims, or
- group (bundle) or ungroup (unbundle) certain MDCs to mesh with their in-house database formatting.

Thus, corporate claims reports may range from as few as 17 MDCs (when bundled) to as many as 25 MDCs (when unbundled). Standard MDCs is the list that is used when neither bundling nor unbundling occurs and when even those categories that contain no claims are included.

Standard MDCs

- Accidents, injuries, and poisoning
- Blood-related
- Burns
- Circulatory
- Congenital and perinatal
- Digestive
- Ear/nose/throat
- Endocrine/nutrition/metabolic (including diabetes)
- Factors influencing health status
- Female reproductive
- Genitourinary
- Injury and poisoning
- Hepatobiliary (liver and gallbladder) and pancreas

(continued)

- Infectious and parasitic
- Mental, drug, and alcohol
- Musculoskeletal
- Neoplasm (cancer)
- Nervous (nervous system disorders)
- Pregnancy
- Respiratory
- Male reproductive
- Signs/symptoms/ill-defined (too vague to clearly warrant a distinct MDC; for example, abdominal pain that has no recognizable cause)
- Skin/subcutaneous

International Classification of Disease and Diagnostic Related Groups

As more employers seek to gain more information from their claims data, it is vital to obtain data beyond the level of major diagnostic categories. Why? Because MDCs are generic classifications and, thus, do not reveal the specific nature of a person's diagnosis, condition, or disease. For example, musculoskeletal is one of the most common MDCs at many worksites. By having MDC claims data that are categorized (itemized) by International Classification of Disease or Diagnostic Related Group, you can identify specific conditions, illnesses, or disabilities, such as muscle strains, bad backs, and sprained ankles. Tables 3.1 and 3.2 illustrate reports provided in the ICD and DRG formats. Though other types of formats are sometimes used, they are not as common as these two and thus will not be covered here.

Table 3.1 Sample ICD Classifications: Outpatient Claims Report

MDC: Musculoskeletal

ICD code	Number of claims	Total charges	Average charge/claim
Arthritis 714.0	105	$47,775	$445
Stiff joint 719.5	13	$11,700	$900
Lumbago 724.2	53	$26,553	$501

Table 3.2 Sample DRG Classifications: Inpatient Claims Report

MDC: Circulatory

DRG number	Number of claims	Total charges	Average charge/claim
Atherosclerosis 132	4	$15,890	$3,972
Hypertension 134	14	$16,000	$1,142
Angina pectoris 140	8	$14,023	$1,752

A CDA Case Study

A claims data analysis can reveal, among many things, the success, failure, or needs of a company's worksite health promotion program. For instance, take a look at three consecutive years of data on a large multihospital chain in the Midwest as shown in table 3.3. The year-to-year patterns reveal a mixture of favorable and unfavorable findings. For example, low back ailments increased significantly in the third year and made up approximately 4% of all employee claims. Breast cancer claims also increased significantly from the previous years and generated heightened awareness by health management personnel. In contrast, hypertension claims declined substantially in the third year as did stress and depression-related claims. Based on these mixed trends, the organization recognized the need to expand and intensify its occupational low back health stretching and flexibility programs, and redesigned its breast cancer screening efforts to target younger women.

Table 3.3 Number of Employees' Claims and As a Percentage of All ICDs (Employees and Dependents)

1997

Rank	ICD	Number of claims	% of total
1	Lung cancer	1,168	2.26
2	Chest pain	826	1.62
3	Hypertension	797	1.54
4	Abdominal pain	719	1.39
5	Stress reaction	712	1.38
6	Systemic lupus	694	1.34
7	Depression	646	1.25
8	Lumbago	638	1.23
9	Diabetes	571	1.10
10	Female menopause	517	1.10

1998

Rank	ICD	Number of claims	% of total
1	Lung cancer	708	1.77
2	Chest pain	706	1.76
3	Hypertension	698	1.73
4	Abdominal pain	675	1.69
5	Stress reaction	569	1.42
6	Back strain	528	1.32
7	Depression	527	1.31
8	Cervical strain	464	1.16
9	Diabetes	423	1.10
10	Female menopause	419	1.0

(continued)

1999			
Rank	**ICD**	**Number of claims**	**% of total**
1	Low back	1,816	3.76
2	Breast cancer	1,653	3.42
3	Gynecological exam	1,521	3.15
4	Chest pain	854	1.77
5	Abdominal pain	812	1.68
6	Hypertension	599	1.24
7	Stress reaction	489	1.00
8	Depression	304	.60
9	Enlarged lymph	302	.60
10	Rhinitis	302	.60

In-House or Not?

Organizations planning to do claims data analysis should first determine if it is feasible to do so in-house. If it is not, they should look to other alternatives.

In-House CDA Requirements

The major requirements for doing an in-house analysis include the following:

- Adequate time for personnel to request, acquire, review, and analyze the data
- Ability to obtain appropriate claims data from insurers, third-party claim administrators (TPAs), or health care providers
- A teamwork approach in which key departmental personnel (benefits, medical, safety, human resources, risk management, etc.) share information about what types of claims data formats they need from the TPA and the uses to which they will put them (this collective input will enable whoever is making the requests to the TPA or insurers to guide those organizations in preparing appropriate claims data reports)
- Well-considered procedures that guide evaluators through a step-by-step process to conduct an analysis effectively (see figure 3.1)
- Personnel who are knowledgeable in risk identification and appraisal techniques if the CDA is going to involve risk identification and appraisal (pages 72-77)

Alternatives to In-House CDA

If you determine that you will be unable to perform the CDA in-house, you still have several options. Consultants, local resources, and grants should all be checked out.

Consultants

Be sure to check with colleagues for referrals. Thoroughly interview the top candidates and solicit feedback from all staff members. An employer should generally ask prospective firms the following questions:

- **Personnel:** What types of credentials does your analytical staff have? How many years have you been in the data analysis business? How do you stay apprised of new developments in the industry? Be sure than any consultant you choose has degrees in an analytical field of study such as math, biostatistics, or epidemiology as well as a minimum of five years of on-the-job experience.

- **Clientele:** What size companies do you generally serve? What size of companies do you prefer to serve, or is a company's size irrelevant to you? Your consultant should have experience with companies of all sizes representing various industries.

- **Data needs:** What types of data do you need to perform a thorough analysis? If only outpatient data are readily available, what strategies do you use to request inpatient data? (See *Phase I*, page 60, for the types of strategies you should look for.) Be wary of any consultant who does not state a preference for MDCs separated by ICD and DRG, employees versus dependents, inpatient versus outpatient. They should have experience with using multiple data sources, including a state-wide hospital database and data from a large insurer or TPA.

- **Analytical process:** Do you use a standard set of procedures in conducting a data analysis? If so, what are they? (See figure 3.1 for an example of acceptable procedures.) What types of analyses do you perform with ICD or DRG data beyond the scope of analyzing MDCs? (See *Phase II, Step One*, page 64.) Do you use the same approach for each project or can you customize a project around a client's particular requests? The potential consultant should be able to describe their analytical framework clearly and to give specific examples of various analyses within their capabilities.

- **Database:** Do you rely on public sector databases, or do you have an in-house proprietary database? If you have an in-house database, what types of data are contained in it? Does it reflect the demographic makeup of your company's population? Does it contain local, state, regional, or national norms? How often do you update the database? Ideally, the consultant should have an in-house database containing data relevant to a client.

- **Analytical methodology:** What analytical methods do you use in conducting a CDA? How are your analytical methods superior to those used by other firms? Can you accurately measure the proportionate influence of certain risk factors (lifestyle, environmental, genetic, health care) on health care utilization and costs? (See *Risk Factor Cost Appraisal*, page 72.) If so, how? Do you conduct medical care cost forecasts? (See chapter 4.) If so, what inflation indices are used and why? Consultants should be able to cite two or three key differences between themselves and their major competitors, and they should be willing to give you names of clients, preferably known to you, who can say something about the accuracy of the consultants' forecasts.

- **Cost:** Is the cost based on a set fee (that is, per project) or hourly charges? Does the quantity or type of data provided influence the cost? How do your per capita (per enrollee) charges compare with the industry norm? Consider the pros and cons of paying a flat project fee versus an hourly fee. Organizations should avoid consultants who ask to be paid up front or do not agree to negotiate a specific number of hours.

- **Quality assurance:** How do you ensure the accuracy (validity) and consistency (reliability) of your analysis? The potential consultant should specify that its methodology has been verified by an outside independent organization and that an in-house peer review is a standard quality assurance mechanism.

- **Processing time:** What was the quickest turnaround time for completing a claims data analysis? Why? What was the longest turnaround time for completing a

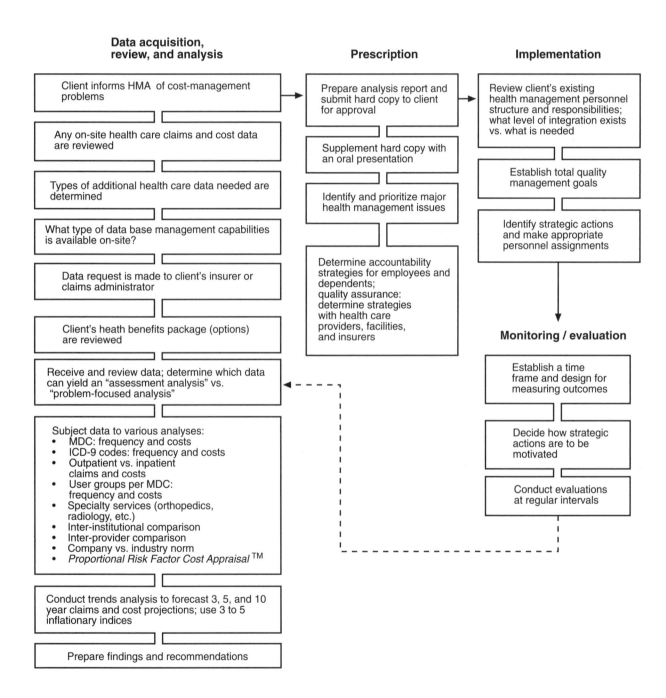

EconoCalc & PRFCA ™

Health Care Claim and Cost Analysis

Data acquisition, review, and analysis

Client informs HMA of cost-management problems

Any on-site health care claims and cost data are reviewed

Types of additional health care data needed are determined

What type of data base management capabilities is available on-site?

Data request is made to client's insurer or claims administrator

Client's heath benefits package (options) are reviewed

Receive and review data; determine which data can yield an "assessment analysis" vs. "problem-focused analysis"

Subject data to various analyses:
- MDC: frequency and costs
- ICD-9 codes: frequency and costs
- Outpatient vs. inpatient claims and costs
- User groups per MDC: frequency and costs
- Specialty services (orthopedics, radiology, etc.)
- Inter-institutional comparison
- Inter-provider comparison
- Company vs. industry norm
- *Proportional Risk Factor Cost Appraisal* ™

Conduct trends analysis to forecast 3, 5, and 10 year claims and cost projections; use 3 to 5 inflationary indices

Prepare findings and recommendations

Prescription

Prepare analysis report and submit hard copy to client for approval

Supplement hard copy with an oral presentation

Identify and prioritize major health management issues

Determine accountability strategies for employees and dependents; quality assurance: determine strategies with health care providers, facilities, and insurers

Implementation

Review client's existing health management personnel structure and responsibilities; what level of integration exists vs. what is needed

Establish total quality management goals

Identify strategic actions and make appropriate personnel assignments

Monitoring / evaluation

Establish a time frame and design for measuring outcomes

Decide how strategic actions are to be motivated

Conduct evaluations at regular intervals

Figure 3.1 A flow chart describing a sample step-by-step process for conducting a claims data analysis.
Copyright 1998, Health Management Associates

claims data analysis? Why? Obtain a sample contract from the top candidates to see how long they believe it will take them to complete the services requested.

• **Final report:** Is your standard report prepared for a particular decision maker, such as a benefits director, safety manager, or occupational health nurse, or is it applicable to all health management personnel? Are you willing to customize a report to include specific graphics (tables and charts) and whether it is printed in black and white, gray tone, or color? Is the report also provided to the client in an electronic format? Does each client receive a disk copy of the report? Consultants should be willing to customize the style and ratio of narrative to illustrations to a client's request.

• **Ancillary resources:** Can you make an on-site presentation of the final report, if requested? If so, at what cost? Can you assist clients in implementing key recommendations from the final reports? If so, do you charge an extra fee? How have you assisted previous clients? Consultants should give examples of how they have provided these services to previous clients.

By formulating relevant questions before hiring an outside vendor, and knowing what answers they are looking for, employers are more likely to choose a firm that produces quality information in terms of both time and money.

Local Resources and Grants

A second option for organizations choosing not to do an in-house claims data analysis is to use local resources. For example, a nearby university may have a professor skilled in the area of claims data analysis who would be interested in doing an analysis for a nominal fee or in exchange for being allowed to use the company as a research site. Perhaps that same university offers a graduate program in statistics or worksite health promotion, and your organization would offer a perfect opportunity for graduate students to try out their developing skills (supervised by a well-qualified professor, of course). Or the local health department may have a biostatistician or epidemiology expert who would be qualified and willing to do a CDA for a nominal fee. Creative brainstorming about the assets in your community may yield a surprising number of options you had not considered before.

Finally, an organization may seek grant monies from a state, regional, or national association to pay for a claims analysis. For example, the Mecklenburg County Health Department used a grant from the local chapter of the American Heart Association to have a claims data analysis conducted on four companies in Charlotte, North Carolina. The analysis was used as a baseline and outcome evaluation of a two-year cardiovascular risk reduction program for the four worksites. A similar approach was taken in New York state where a grant from the New York State Physical Activity Coalition provided monies for a medical claims analysis of the state government's health care costs.

CDA Phase I

Once you have determined who is going to do your claims data analysis (pages 57-60), you must plan the CDA. One reasonable way to organize a claims data analysis is shown in *Suggested Steps for CDA*. In this section we examine Phase I in some detail. The following two sections discuss Phases II and III.

Suggested Steps for CDA

A practical claims data analysis strategy consists of the following steps:

- **Phase I**
  1. Access and review existing on-site claims reports.
  2. Develop goals for an analysis.
- **Phase II**
  1. Formulate questions for requesting data.
  2. Having obtained the data, begin review.
- **Phase III**
  1. Analyze data.
  2. Identify key trends and challenges.
  3. Develop a report for key decision makers.

Phase I, Step One: Access and Review Existing On-Site Claims Reports

Although most companies receive claims reports from their third party administrator (TPA) or insurer, various factors influence the quality of what they get:

- TPAs/insurers stand to make less profit from smaller companies, so the little guys are sometimes viewed less favorably than larger organizations and thus are often overlooked. Therefore, if you are a smaller company, you must be prepared to be the squeaky wheel.

- An organization is more likely to receive claims data if these reports are positioned as a standard benefit of their contract with the insurer/TPA. You should look over your company's contract with your insurer/TPA and ask the responsible parties to renegotiate if claims data reports are not mandated.

- An organization is also more likely to receive claims data if their TPA/insurer has an efficient claims data management system in place. If you find that current claims data reports are not satisfactory, find out from the TPA/insurer what sort of claims data management system they use. If their system is deficient, ask what their plans are to upgrade. If they have no plans, again, speak to the responsible parties in your company about working with the TPA/insurer to improve their systems. Otherwise, consider switching providers.

- Finally, if a TPA/insurer has a strong customer-service orientation, it is more likely to provide its clients with annual claims data reports. Again, if your provider is unwilling or unable to give you the kind of service you ask for, even after targeted discussions and a reasonable amount of time for change, ask your company to look into different providers.

Even though most companies are given some kind of claims reports by their TPA/insurer, surveys indicate that less than 50% actually analyze their data. There is no point in having data unless you plan to do something with it. The first thing to do is to determine if key claims data are missing. Some major tip-offs that this is the case include the following:

- Little or no utilization data. The number of claims are not listed.
- Little or no charge or payment data. No dollar amounts are provided.
- No distinction between inpatient and outpatient claims, charges, and payments.
- No distinction between employees' and dependents' claims, charges, and payments.
- Vaguely described claim categories: MDCs, ICDs, or DRGs are not identified by name descriptions or numerical codes.

What Were They Thinking?

Imagine that a midsized semiconductor manufacturing firm in the Northeast, which offered two plans to its 500 employees and covered dependents (HMO and PPO), wished to conduct a claims data analysis to answer the following questions:

- What are the most common types of claims?
- What are the fastest-growing claims?
- What are the most expensive types of claims?
- What percentage of total claims are incurred by employees? By dependents?
- What potentially modifiable risk factors are costing the organization the most?

The data supplied by their health claims administrator are shown in table 3.4.

Table 3.4 Amounts Paid by Type of Claim and Place of Service

	Institutional		Professional	
Inpatient	Ancillary	$395,173	Surgery	$82,845
	Room/board	$123,691	Medical care	$34,863
			Anesthesia	$17,790
			Assisted surgery	$ 2,178
Outpatient	Ancillary	$132,460	Surgery	$32,442
			Radiology	$11,333
			Medical care	$13,564
			Anesthesia	$ 3,094
			Pathology	$ 2,370
			Laboratory	$ 3,238
			All others	$ 21
Office			Medical care	$49,516
			Surgery	$35,696
			Radiology	$30,445
			Laboratory	$46,751
			Physical therapy	$ 4,028
			Dentistry	$ 2,112
Other	Home health	$ 1,158	Medical supplies	$ 711
	All others	$ 398	Orthopedic appliance	$ 1,029
			All others	$ 2,255
Total		$652,880		$376,281

(continued)

Upon scanning this report, the company was dismayed to realize that the data did not address the questions they had posed. Before you read what the company did, list on a piece of paper what further information you would ask the health claims administrator to provide. Once you have listed your questions, continue reading and compare your answer with what the company, in fact, did.

After analyzing the report's deficiencies, health managers requested the following additional data:

- Diagnostic categories, including MDCs, ICDs, and DRGs
- Utilization information including both the overall number of health care visits and utilization by delivery site (inpatient versus outpatient)
- Enrollee utilization and payments by employees and by dependents
- Plan-specific information, distinguishing HMO data from PPO data.

As a result of identifying these deficiencies, senior management representatives met with the health plan administrators and mutually configured a more informative format for future claims data reports.

Phase I, Step Two: Develop Goals for an Analysis

There are two primary ways for developing goals for a claims data analysis. The first is to develop goals before you look at claims data. For instance, an organization may decide to develop and use the following generic goals before it reviews claims data:

- Compare the five most common types of claims this year versus last year, as a percentage of total claims.
- Compare the five most expensive types of claims this year versus last year, as a percentage of total charges.
- Identify the number of employees filing at least three claims this year versus last year.
- Compare average per capita health care charges for employees this year versus last year.

A second and more strategic way to establish goals for a claims analysis is to first perform a preliminary review of claims data, then use the resulting information to establish the specific goals of the more comprehensive evaluation. For example, if an organization's claims utilization rate rose 20% and charges rose 25%, that information suggests the following **data-driven goals:**

- Identify the major types of claims that represent a disproportionately high percentage of all claims, such as circulatory, neoplasm, or digestive.
- Identify the five most expensive types of ICD or DRG conditions within the two most expensive MDCs.
- Identify the five fastest-growing ICDs and DRGs by number of claims over the past three years.
- Identify the five fastest-growing ICDs and DRGs by charges over the past three years.

The questions asked in CDA (and thus, its goals) should be based not only on what is suggested by a preliminary review of the data but also on the interests of key decision makers. For example, a benefits manager may be particularly interested in using claims data to compare health plan costs from year to year; an occupational health nurse may be interested in monitoring the prevalence of on-the-job back injuries; and the health promotion program director may be interested in whether or not the employees-only fitness center use policy is reducing the prevalence of circulatory claims more in employees than in dependents. If the data, personnel, and hours are available to deal with all these questions, they should become goals of the evaluation.

CDA Phase II

Once you have determined what data are available in-house and what the goals of your evaluation are going to be, you can proceed to Phase II . This phase will involve formulating questions to ask your TPA/insurer if you need additional data and reviewing the data once they arrive.

Phase II, Step One: Formulate Questions for Requesting Additional Data

Although, as noted above, most midsized and large organizations receive some type of health care claims data reports from their insurers or TPAs on an annual basis, many of these reports are long on numbers and short on information. Traditionally, organizations have asked only **basic assessment** questions when requesting claims data reports, such as the following:

- What are the most common types of claims?
- What are the most expensive types of claims?
- What is the average length of stay for the most common (inpatient) conditions?
- How do this year's total charges compare with last year's charges?

The answers to such generic questions will provide the employer with some strategic planning value. But that value is limited. How can you know what questions to ask to obtain more useful data? These six areas will give you some clues: the composition of your enrollee population; inpatient versus outpatient issues; expense by type of claim; factors influencing health levels; annual data over several years; and data on external populations.

- **Enrollee subgroups:** If your organization provides health care benefits to dependents and retirees, be sure to request claims data reports that include all enrolled groups. This level of specificity will reveal differences between and within each of the enrollee groups. For example, a typical profile may highlight the following differences:

Group	% of enrollees	% of claims	% of costs
Employees	40%	30%	25%
Spouse dependents	50%	50%	45%
Child dependents	10%	20%	30%

- **Outpatient versus inpatient:** Typically, an organization may have an outpatient-to-inpatient claims ratio in the neighborhood of 80% to 20%, yet the ratio of inpatient charges to outpatient charges may be as close as, say, 60% to 40%. Why are these differences so disproportionately large? Because outpatient claims are considerably less expensive than the inpatient claims. For example, a hypertensive condition treated in an outpatient setting may cost no more than several hundred dollars including the cost of medication. However, a more serious hypertensive condition requiring an overnight hospital (inpatient) stay may cost several thousand dollars when figuring in room and board, ancillary services, physician charges, and medication. Thus, outpatient versus inpatient comparisons—in addition to employees versus dependents comparisons—can be used by benefits, human resources, risk management, safety, and occupational health managers to guide their planning efforts.

• **Expense by type of claim:** No two claim categories share the same percentage of an organization's health care costs. Although there may be some cost similarity among, say, the top five or six MDCs, it is not uncommon to see significant cost differences between these top categories. Moreover, it's important to realize that even claims categories with a small percentage of total claims can still account for a significant portion of an organization's total health care costs. This is particularly true for categories such as neoplasm (cancer), mental health, congenital, blood-related, and digestive conditions. To some extent, circulatory and nervous categories also show this pattern.

• **Factors influencing health levels:** Since various factors influence a person's overall health status, it is important to subject claims data to a risk factor cost appraisal (described later in this chapter). This type of appraisal can reveal the most expensive risk factors as well as the factors (lifestyle, genetics, environment, etc.) that most strongly influence them.

• **Annual data over several years:** Having several consecutive years of data provides a representative profile of employees' health care utilization and cost patterns. Likewise, an accurate baseline provides a solid foundation on which to conduct progress evaluations at designated intervals throughout an intervention. This benchmark also enhances the accuracy of forecasting.

• **Data on external populations:** Many organizations want to compare their health care utilization and cost patterns against others nationwide or against such patterns in their region, industry, or state. Due to growing pressure from their corporate clients, a growing number of insurers and TPAs are reformatting their corporate claims reports to provide some of these comparative measures.

You can see, then, that to get the data, you need to understand the scope and details of an organization's health care utilization and cost patterns. To spot future trends, you should ask **problem-focused** questions such as the following:

• What are the most common claims by MDC, ICD, and DRG?

• What are the most expensive types of claims by MDC, ICD, and DRG?

• How does our outpatient utilization rate compare with local, regional, and national norms?

• What have our fastest-growing types of outpatient claims been in the past five years?

• What percentage of total health care charges for the top five outpatient MDCs were incurred by employees? Spouses? Dependent children?

• What percentage of charges for the top five inpatient ICDs are linked to lifestyle? Environmental and occupational factors? Genetics? Poor health care? Gender?

• What has the annual cost for each MDC, IDC, and DRG been over the past four years?

• How do our per capita (per enrollee) charges compare with the industry norm?

Phase II, Step Two: Having Obtained the Data, Begin Review

Once your TPA/insurer has responded to your request for additional data, you must review them to confirm that you have received everything that you asked for. Go over the questions you asked during the previous step and be sure that you have a report that applies to each. Also ask the following: *Are the data properly formatted by MDC, ICD, or DRG? Are there separate inpatient and outpatient data reports? Is there a clear distinction between employees' claims and dependents' claims?* If the answer to any of the preceding questions is *no*, or if your TPA/insurer reports do not include everything you asked for, request the delineated reports you need once again. If your TPA/insurer is not used to supplying this level of detail to your company, you may find that it will take more than one try to get what you want from them. Once you have established your insistence that you must have what you've asked for, you'll find that most TPAs/insurers will respond to future requests from you more quickly.

CDA Phase III

Now that you have laid the groundwork for your claims data analysis, you can proceed to the core of the procedure—analyzing the data and reporting your conclusions.

Phase III, Step One: Analyze Data

What does it mean to analyze data? Analysis involves identifying relevant data, then breaking that data down or organizing it in meaningful ways.

Identify Relevant Data

To identify the relevant data, you must revisit your goals and the questions that generated them. For instance, suppose an organization wants to conduct CDA to identify the most expensive risk factors so it can create health promotion programs targeted at high-risk employees. In this case, analysis would be confined to employee-based claims. Or suppose the organization wants to determine if the strong interest in mental health programs that employees expressed on a recent survey is related to the company's health care utilization patterns. To answer that question, an organization could examine its employee-based claims related to anxiety, depression, and post-traumatic stress to see if the level of these stress-related claims is also high, indicating some kind of correlation between employees expressed interests and the problems they take to health care providers.

Analyze Relevant Data

If you were asked to describe CDA in one sentence, you might say that it is asking the right questions to generate necessary reports based on health care claims, then organizing and manipulating the appropriate data from those reports to answer those right questions.

Suppose, for example, that management at your company is interested in knowing if there were any substantial changes from one year to the next in health care utilization and charges over the past three years. To answer this question, you have obtained the claims data listed in table 3.5. You could begin your analysis by reviewing the data in a chronological sequence (1998, 1999, and 2000). Using the chronological approach, the first step would be to identify the most common MDCs in 1998, then in 1999, and finally in 2000. Your organization's MDC utilization rankings based on the data in table 3.5 are as follows:

Computer Tip

Many insurers and TPAs prepare corporate claims data reports in a spreadsheet format. These formats contain rows and columns of data which are separated by MDCs, ICDs, or DRGs. In-house health management personnel who are familiar with spreadsheet layouts and formulas can easily compute sums, means (averages), and other outcome measures for a CDA using these formats. If you aren't familiar with this process, access the Help feature in your computer to learn about various ways to do basic spreadsheet computations.

Rank	1998	1999	2000
1st	Musculoskeletal	Ill-defined	Musculoskeletal
2nd	Ill-defined	Musculoskeletal	Ill-defined
3nd	Factors influencing health status	Factors influencing health status	Circulatory
4th	Circulatory	Circulatory	Factors influencing health status
5th	Genitourinary	Genitourinary	Genitourinary

You will note little variability in the top five claim categories from year to year. This degree of consistency is very common in typical workforces because people tend to use health care services for similar reasons from one year to the next.

Are there other changes (or lack thereof) that you could spot from table 3.5? Yes. You could, for example, identify changes in the cost of the various MDCs. Unlike utilization rankings, which tend to vary little from year to year, claims charges can, and often do, vary considerably in a short time frame. One reason is that an unexpectedly high number of catastrophic medical claims, or even a single catastrophic claim such as an organ transplant, can significantly increase the overall charges for a particular MDC. Note that neoplasm charges increased 250% from 1998 to 2000 despite a mere 17% increase in neoplasm claims. Why? If you were to request further data in this case, you would discover that it was because of a higher percentage of high-cost catastrophic cancer claims.

Table 3.5   Outpatient Claims and Charges by MDC

MDC	1998 Number	1998 Charges ($)	1999 Number	1999 Charges ($)	2000 Number	2000 Charges ($)
Circulatory	726	700,500	800	900,900	850	950,100
Musculoskeletal	900	700,900	905	740,890	930	800,980
Neoplasms	150	380,010	157	856,890	176	950,900
Ill-defined	789	300,500	908	340,789	890	375,908
Digestive	349	605,670	389	670,900	400	710,980
Genitourinary	450	235,345	701	237,453	459	287,890
Injury/poisoning	101	67,890	105	70,890	109	72,345
Respiratory	356	208,980	300	175,989	250	135,098
Factors	780	349,908	767	343,890	756	324,230
Nervous	45	23,456	57	29,976	60	34,564
Pregnancy	25	76,005	35	89,786	27	79,997
Perinatal	5	4,989	6	7,678	4	7,890
Mental	95	67,890	98	76,976	99	77,989
Endocrine/metabolic	80	46,897	82	48,987	88	56,789
Infectious	32	4,909	33	5,210	28	4,399
Congenital	2	4,890	1	3,980	2	5,321
Skin/subcutaneous	14	6,780	15	7,234	17	8,899
Blood-related	3	3,450	4	5,990	2	3,567
External injury	45	12,459	47	13,879	43	11,876

Yet another change that could be identified with this table is which MDC has been the fastest growing over the past three years. The data tell us that the fourth-highest MDC, circulatory, actually increased more (35%) than any other MDC from 1998 to 2000. This statistic can be identified as a **trend** because a measurable variable (utilization) experienced a consistent increase, decrease, or stability over a specified time frame. Most of the MDCs in table 3.5 showed an upward trend in both utilization and charges. Yet, there was a substantial year-to-year decrease in respiratory claims.

Since there is usually variability in year-to-year charge rankings, it is necessary to analyze data over several years to identify a legitimate trend. As a result of the preceding utilization and charge comparisons, the analyst can identify outcomes, trends, and challenges to include in the final report. (Chapter 6 discusses how to prepare such reports.)

These data could also be used to spot the MDCs that were most commonly the subject of claims for the past three years:

Rank	MDC	Three-year sum of total claims
1st	Musculoskeletal	2,735
2nd	Ill-defined	2,587
3rd	Circulatory	2,376
4th	Factors influencing health status	2,303
5th	Genitourinary	1,610

It is clear that musculoskeletal claims were the most common MDC over the three-year time frame. Although this information indicates that targeting musculoskeletal disorders in your WHP programming is probably a good idea, you need to evaluate other factors to confirm that. If you consider only the total number of claims in an MDC, you could end up targeting an area that is too broad (such as ill-defined) to have much of an impact on. Or you could fail to target a group that has very few, but very expensive claims, such as endocrine/nutrition/metabolic, and whose health could be very positively impacted by relatively inexpensive interventions such as diabetes education or support groups.

Practice Analyses

The following are short sections from three kinds of reports that are typically generated by looking at claims. By considering some of the questions listed under *Phase II, Step One,* and looking at the data in tables 3.6, 3.7, and 3.8, you can see how the numbers provided in such reports can be used to answer specific questions.

1. Table 3.6 shows an annual group summary of claims and payments by MDC. Evaluators can analyze these data in several ways, such as

   • By determining the highest number of claims by MDC for employees versus dependents

   • By determining the highest-ranking payments by MDC for employees versus dependents

   • By comparing male employees versus male dependents and female employees versus female dependents on claims and payments by MDC

   • By comparing total number of claims for employees versus dependents by gender to determine a per capita average (the number of employees and dependents are needed for this comparison).

Run each of these analyses on the data in table 3.6 and compare your results with others.

(continued)

	Employee male		Employee female		Dependent male		Dependent female	
MDC	**Claims (#)**	**Paid ($)**	**Claims (#)**	**Paid ($)**	**Claims (#)**	**Paid ($)**	**Claims (#)**	**Paid ($)**
Circulatory	454	197,252	1,677	609,809	1,274	572,949	160	88,763
Musculoskeletal	725	240,093	4,254	681,083	911	252,488	695	131,134
Neoplasms	133	28,095	2,668	866,231	687	338,795	388	76,710
Ill-defined	465	82,968	3,638	703,596	712	165,133	557	107,516
Digestive	217	133,525	1,335	762,858	229	108,395	149	55,584
Genitourinary	161	24,538	1,981	702,944	396	182,809	273	92,411
Injury/poison	198	101,526	1,583	491,662	387	90,381	155	38,391
Respiratory	226	59,930	1,563	379,086	543	130,143	301	63,613
Health status	186	25,766	4,409	364,822	451	115,791	759	36,548
Nervous	123	27,888	964	181,469	143	35,916	297	51,704
Pregnancy	0	0	524	300,973	0	0	175	73,675
Mental	314	28,549	1,581	176,602	121	10,621	264	16,396
Endocrine	229	18,898	1,189	147,411	409	51,587	207	13,493
Infectious	58	7,228	287	64,979	62	41,856	45	12,840
Congenital	19	8,418	48	26,026	8	27,484	5	482
Perinatal	0	0	4	2,383	2	157	3	1,620
Skin/subcutaneous	65	6,147	405	25,255	69	16,953	70	3,682
Blood disease	11	728	169	15,649	62	6,290	51	2,105
External injury	0	0	11	1,348	0	0	0	0
Total	3,584	991,549	28,290	6,504,186	6,466	2,147,798	4,554	866,667

Table 3.6 An Annual Group Summary of Claims and Payments by Major Diagnostic Category (MDC)

2. The data in table 3.7 can be subjected to the same types of analyses used to interpret the numbers in table 3.6. However, this report also enables evaluators to analyze and compare specific illnesses and conditions rather than confining themselves to broadly defined categories. For example, high blood pressure is the most common circulatory claim, and it can be addressed in various worksite health management interventions— for example, expanding hypertension screening from older employees to younger employees (or to all employees) on a regular basis and offering financial incentives for participating in customized exercise, nutrition, and stress management programs. Some of the questions you could answer by looking at this report include the following: Do employees file more or fewer claims than dependents? Which conditions are more common in each group? What are the most expensive types of claims on average overall, and, in each group? Answer these questions using the data in table 3.7 and discuss your results with others.

3. The data in table 3.8 allow evaluators to perform some of the comparisons previously described in addition to comparing specific DRGs by the **average length of stay**

(continued)

(continued)

(ALOS). These data reveal the most serious conditions, which warrant longer periods of stay, and their associated expenses. The paid column reflects the amount paid by the employer. Any difference between charges and amount paid is usually paid by the employee (patient) through their out-of-pocket deductible and co-payment. What are the most serious conditions listed in table 3.8, and why do you suspect they are more serious than other conditions? Although medical back problems appear to be the most common inpatient claim, they represent about one-half the average length of stay for septic arthritis. What factors might explain this discrepancy? Perform these analyses and compare your findings with others.

Table 3.7   An Abbreviated Sample of Annual Outpatient Claims by Circulatory International Classification of Disease (ICD)

		Employees		Dependents	
ICD code	Description	Claims (#)	Paid ($)	Claims (#)	Paid ($)
401	Essential hypertension	14	7,345	13	6,897
412	Old myocardial infarction	2	14,890	3	17,687
414	Chronic ischemic heart disease	4	10,898	1	4,345
419	Bacterial infection	1	4,865	0	0
420	Acute pericarditis	2	8,901	1	4,501
425	Cardiomyopathy	2	18,768	1	9,675
431	Intracerebral hemorrhage	1	14,989	2	30,969
436	Cerebrovascular accident	2	15,678	2	17,891
448	Disease, capillaries	1	4,567	2	7,989

Table 3.8   An Abbreviated Sample Report of Inpatient Musculoskeletal Claims and Payments by Diagnostic-Related Group (DRG)

DRG	Description	Admissions	Days	ALOS	Charges ($)	Paid ($)
235	Fractures of femur	2	4	2	15,000	12,500
238	Osteomyelitis	2	6	3	14,890	11,899
242	Septic arthritis	4	24	6	12,897	10,980
243	Med. back problems	9	28	3.1	23,005	19,670
244	Arthropathies w/cc	3	10	3.1	15,908	14,905
245	Arthropathies w/o cc	3	3	1	10,900	8,900
248	Tendonitis, bursitis	5	5	1	2,345	1,500
249	Aftercare	2	4	2	12,908	10,980

Phase III, Step Two: Reporting Your Conclusions

When reporting your CDA conclusions, you must again consider who your stakeholders are and address the concerns of each individual or subgroup within that larger group. It may be appropriate to do separate reports for each of these, or it may be advantageous to do one large report with clearly targeted sections. Since the point of doing assessment is to see if programs are on the right track—and if not, why—you must include appropriate recommendations and be prepared to assist in implementing them. Chapter 6 discusses at length how to create and present reports of all kinds.

Considering Common Outcomes

When reviewing MDCs, claims data analysts will find that certain outcomes are usual in many categories. Some of these outcomes include the following:

- **Accidents, injury, and poisoning:** Physical trauma, frostbite, heat conditions, and other conditions are common in heavy labor and high-risk occupations.

- **Circulatory:** These claims are especially common in male-oriented workforces and typically rank high in overall charges.

- **Digestive:** Common in most worksites, some conditions—polyps, in particular—suggest an increased risk for colorectal cancer.

- **Factors influencing health status (FIHS):** This category includes preventive services (well-baby care and immunizations), emergency department visits, laboratory services, and prescription medication.

- **Male reproductive:** Prostate conditions are especially common in workers over 50 years old.

- **Mental:** This condition includes neuroses (e.g., acute depression) and psychoses (e.g., schizophrenia); drug-related conditions may also be coded in this MDC.

- **Musculoskeletal:** Often the most common claim, it is especially common in weekend warriors, dissatisfied workers, and workforces with high-risk occupations.

- **Neoplasm (cancer):** Also referred to as myeloproliferative. Although not that common, individual claims can be very costly.

Although most of the preceding MDCs are common or expensive in many organizations from year to year—making it relatively easy to track and measure annual claims and costs—you should not assume that health care utilization and cost patterns will be similar for all organizations. For example, claims data at one worksite reviewed by the author revealed that nearly 40% of all charges were tied to only three (of 17) MDCs. Nearly 50% of the claims filed at another worksite were confined to only four MDCs. Claims charges in the former organization were largely incurred from a high number of expensive inpatient claims tied to circulatory, cancer, and digestive ailments. In contrast, the other organization had many employees with a disproportionately high number of claims in two (musculoskeletal and factors influencing health status) of the four most prevalent MDCs. Thus, the importance of analyzing each organization's claims data without making assumptions about what you will find is clear.

REVIEW QUESTIONS: CLAIMS DATA ANALYSIS

1. Describe how health management personnel can use a CDA as a front-end prescription and as a back-end evaluation tool.
2. What are three ways in which to classify medical claims data?
3. What are the major requirements for doing an in-house CDA?
4. Describe the steps involved in conducting a CDA.

Risk Factor Cost Appraisal

A **risk factor** can be defined as a biological, behavioral, or occupational attribute or occurrence that increases an individual's risk of premature illness, disability, or death. Risk factors play a significant role in WHP evaluation, and their influence on economics is discussed in the following section.

The Economic Significance of Risk Factors

Many organizations consider **risk factor cost appraisal** to be a key part of their claims data analysis because it reveals the most expensive risk factors in a workforce. This knowledge will help an organization determine the most appropriate health promotion and risk-reduction programs.

A Matter of Risk

A risk factor cost appraisal conducted for a large hospital in the Midwest indicated the following risk factor ranking:

Rank	Risk factor
1st	Physical inactivity
2nd	Obesity
3rd	Family history/genetics
4th	No prework stretching and warm-up
5th	Age > 35
6th	Poor diet
7th	High stress
8th	No job rotation
9th	Cigarette smoking
10th	Diabetes

Of the ten most expensive risk factors, all but two (family history and age > 35), were potentially modifiable by changes in lifestyle, environment, or work style. Armed with this knowledge, program planners targeted their resources and efforts toward lowering the risk factors present in their workforce. For example, the hospital established an in-house walking course and approved a policy to extend lunch breaks an additional 15 minutes for employees who chose to walk during this time frame. In addition, they established a five-minute prework stretch session on work time for all employees. At the quarterly evaluation, risk factor prevalence rates for physical inactivity, stress, and cigarette smoking had dropped an average of 15% among participants.

An organization's risk factor cost profile is also useful for helping WHP management know how to tailor the job descriptions of their personnel to identify and reduce specific risk factors. For example, here are examples of the tasks for which various people involved in WHP may use risk factor cost information:

- Health promotion personnel develop specific lifestyle modification programs.
- Personnel directors design pre-employment job placement criteria.
- Medical workers develop risk factor-specific screenings.
- Human resources staff offer work/life quality enhancement activities.

(continued)

- Benefits employees create financial incentives for healthy habits.
- Safety personnel target high-risk areas for accidents.
- Fitness center staff develop low back flexibility stations.
- Employee assistance workers offer personalized stress management.
- Risk management personnel create integrated risk factor identification systems.

According to the U.S. Department of Health and Human Services and other research organizations, a person's overall risk factor status is influenced significantly by lifestyle, environment, genetics, and health care. The most widely accepted statistics suggest the following:

- **Lifestyle factors** contribute about 51% to one's health risk (e.g., exercise habits, diet, stress level, and tobacco and alcohol use).
- **Environmental factors** contribute about 20% (e.g., occupation and environmental exposures).
- **Genetic factors** account for about 19% (e.g., family's history of certain conditions and diseases).
- **Health care factors** contribute about 10% to one's health risk (e.g., quality of care, diagnostic accuracy).

Since approximately 71% of one's health risk is contributed by lifestyle and environmental factors alone, and since both of these have the potential to be heavily influenced by employers, it is not surprising that organizations are very interested in knowing how much these risk factors are costing them.

The Proportionate Risk Factor Cost Appraisal Technique

Various commercial and proprietary tools have been developed to measure the financial cost of risk factors in an organization. The author uses a risk factor appraisal form known as *Proportionate Risk Factor Cost Appraisal* (PRFCA) to help students and practitioners conduct a risk factor cost analysis once they reach the level of types of claims that are defined by specific MDCs or ICDs (see figure 3.2).

You can subject data to risk factor cost appraisal as long as

- the data are tied to specific MDCs or ICDs,
- claims and cost data are known,
- tangible risk factors can be identified, and
- risk factor weights are known or can be generated.

PRFCA: Steps One and Two

If you have requested claims data from your insurer or TPA properly, you will already have the data you need to perform a proportionate risk factor cost analysis. But if you have not already done so, your first step must be to obtain that data, being sure to request information from the past two or three years on the most common and the most expensive MDCs, ICDs, and DRGs. (As discussed earlier, the most common claims in an organization are usually different from the most expensive claims.) Step two is to determine the five most common and the five most expensive MDCs, and the three most common and the three most expensive ICDs and DRGs within each MDC.

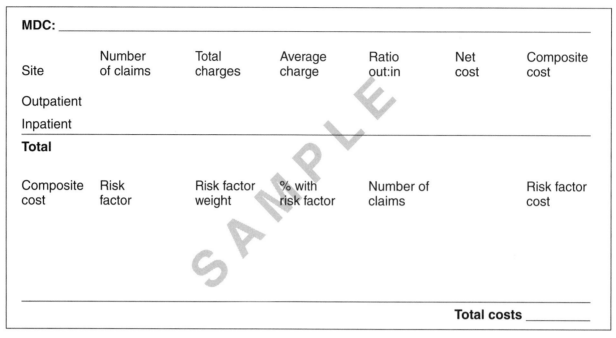

Figure 3.2 A blank Proportionate Risk Factor Cost Appraisal. PRFCA is a registered trademark of Health Management Associates. PRFCA materials contained in this book are provided for educational use only; commercial usage prohibited.

PRFCA: Step Three

The third step involves preparing the upper portion of the cost appraisal form for each ICD or DRG selected by counting, adding, or calculating certain things and recording the results. The following are step-by-step instructions on how to do this. The data are from figure 3.3.

Counting, Adding, and Recording

Count and record the

- number of inpatient claims per ICD, then the
- number of outpatient claims per ICD.

Next, add and record the

- total inpatient charges per ICD, then the
- total outpatient charges per ICD.

The results of this step using the data from figure 3.3 are shown in figure 3.4. You can see that the upper half of the PRFCA has been filled in by simply transplanting the total number of claims and total charges listed in figure 3.3.

Calculating and Recording

Calculate and record the following:

- Average inpatient charge for the group of selected ICDs by dividing total inpatient charges ($34,942) by total number of inpatient claims (7):

$$\frac{\$34,942}{7} = \$4,991$$

MDC: Circulatory

Outpatient

ICD	Number of claims	Payments	Average payment per claim
Hypertension	28	$12,490	$ 446
Ischemia	4	4,791	1,197
Phlebitis	9	9,408	1,045
Total	**41**	**$26,689**	**$ 651**

Inpatient

ICD	Number of admissions	Payments	Average payment/admission
Hypertension	5	$13,470	$ 2,694
Ischemic heart disease	2	21,472	10,736
Total	**7**	**$34,942**	**$ 4,991**

Figure 3.3   A sample data sheet showing several circulatory-based ICDs.

MDC: Circulatory

ICDs (3): Hypertension, ischemia, phlebitis

Site	Number of claims	Total charges	Average charge	Ratio out/in	Net cost	Composite cost
Outpatient	41	$26,689	$ 651	.643	$ 418	$1,099
Inpatient	7	$34,942	$4,991	.357	$1,781	
Total	**48**	**$61,631**				

Composite cost	Risk factor	Risk factor weight	% with risk factor	Number of claims	Risk factor cost

Figure 3.4   A sample PRFCA with completed upper half.
Courtesy of Health Management Associates.

- Average outpatient charges for the group of selected ICDs by dividing total outpatient charges ($26,689) by total number of outpatient claims (41):

$$\frac{\$26,689}{41} = \$651$$

- Outpatient-to-inpatient ratio by computing the percentage of outpatient-to-inpatient claims (.854% to .146%) and the percentage of outpatient-to-inpatient charges (.433% to .567%), then by adding the outpatient percentages together (.854 + .433). Divide by two (2) to determine the outpatient ratio numerator

(.643), then subtract the outpatient ratio numerator (.643) from 1.0 to determine the inpatient denominator (.357).

$$.854 + .433 = \frac{1.287}{2} = .643$$
$$1.00 - .643 = .357$$

- Net cost (for both types of claims) by multiplying average outpatient charge ($651) by outpatient ratio numerator (.643) to determine net outpatient cost ($418) and multiplying average inpatient charge ($4,991) by inpatient ratio denominator (.357) to determine net inpatient cost ($1,781).

$$\$651 \times .643 = \$418$$

$$\$4,991 \times .357 = \$1,781$$

- Composite cost—this is the adjusted/weighted cost of all inpatient and outpatient claims based on the (a) disproportionately higher number of outpatient claims and (b) disproportionately higher average cost of inpatient claims. Add the outpatient net cost ($418) to the inpatient net cost ($1,781) and divide by two to determine the composite cost ($1,099).

$$\$418 + \$1,781 = \$2,199$$

$$\frac{\$2,199}{2} = \$1,099$$

PRFCA: Step Four

The fourth step is to prepare the bottom half of the PRFCA form (figure 3.5) column-by-column:

- In the first column, list the composite cost.
- In the second column, list risk factors associated with the selected ICD. You can find these risk factors in resources such as journals, conference proceedings, professional associations, and databases. Some of these resources are listed in the appendix (pages 189-192).

- In the third column, list the risk factor weight for each risk factor. Each risk factor weight reflects the approximate influence that each risk factor has on the ICD. The maximum weight is 1.0 (100%). For example, a risk factor weight of .15 signifies that 15% of the total risk is due to that particular risk factor. Risk factor weights are based on research studies of public and private-sector worksites. Risk factor weights may be obtained from the professional literature, selected professional associations, and consulting firms who specialize in particular risk factor areas. Many of these resources are listed in the appendix.

- In the fourth column, list the percentage of workers with a specific risk factor. You can find the risk factor prevalence rates in your workforce from various sources. For example, in many worksites the occupational health nurse can provide information on the percentage of employees with specific risk factors. You may also consider employees' feedback from a

Computer Tip

A growing volume of research is available on the Internet as more professional journals and associations have begun to take advantage of this new technology. When searching for information on a particular risk factor, try limiting your search to no more than a few words at a time. Use search words that specifically reflect the scope of your search. For example, if you are searching for a list of cardiovascular risk factors, type in only *cardiovascular risk factors*. This helps the search engines to identify pertinent Web sites quickly.

health risk appraisal (HRA) or other instrument. HRA data alone, however, should not be the sole resource used to gauge risk factor prevalence because it relies primarily on self-reported information. Another resource commonly used to gauge risk factor prevalence is the Behavioral Risk Factor Surveillance Survey (BRFSS), which is a randomized, state-wide survey conducted every two years by the Centers for Disease Control and Prevention (CDC). Check with your local health department or state health department for a copy of your state's BRFSS. Finally, check with your county health department, which may have tracked risk factor prevalence rates in the community. (Employees' risk factor prevalence often reflects that of their community.)

- In the fifth column, list the number of claims for the selected ICD.
- Finally, compute the risk factor cost by multiplying each of the columns.

MDC: Circulatory

ICDs (3): Hypertension, ischemia, phlebitis

Site	Number of claims	Total charges	Average charge	Ratio out/in	Net cost	Composite cost
Outpatient	41	$26,689	$ 651	.643	$ 418	$1,099
Inpatient	7	$34,942	$4,991	.357	$1,781	
Total	**48**	**$61,631**				

Composite cost	Risk factor	Risk factor weight	% with risk factor	Number of claims	Risk factor cost
$1,099	Diabetes	0.18	0.062	48	$ 588
$1,099	Obesity	0.17	0.350	48	3,138
$1,099	Smoking	0.14	0.250	48	1,846
$1,099	Inactivity	0.12	0.600	48	3,798
$1,099	Hypertension	0.12	0.210	48	1,329
$1,099	High cholesterol	0.11	0.200	48	1,160
$1,099	Alcohol abuse	0.05	0.070	48	184
$1,099	Depression	0.04	0.050	48	105
$1,099	Family history	0.04	0.100	48	211
$1,099	Age >40	0.03	0.250	48	395
				Total	**$12,754**

Figure 3.5 A sample PRFCA with completed lower half.
Courtesy of Health Management Associates.

REVIEW QUESTIONS: RISK FACTOR COST APPRAISAL

1. What is the primary reason for doing a risk factor cost appraisal?
2. What factors primarily influence a person's overall risk factor status?
3. What are the major steps involved in conducting a risk factor cost appraisal?

CHAPTER REVIEW

Summary

The two non-econometric data analysis tools described in this chapter (CDA and risk factor cost appraisal) provide worksite health management personnel with specific ready-to-use instruments to track and measure various types of basic data. Despite their straightforward nature, both tools give decision makers a relative degree of flexibility to tailor their analytical approaches around an organization's claims data and risk factor profile. Specifically, CDA can identify an organization's most common and most expensive claims and costs and thus reveal the most pressing employee health and cost-containment challenges at hand. Likewise, risk factor cost appraisal can generate the type of data needed to establish a strong prescription to guide decision makers in their programming decisions. Once these tools have been implemented at a worksite, health management personnel can proceed with econometric analysis tools such as break-even analysis, cost-effectiveness analysis, benefit-cost analysis, and forecasting. Each of these tools is presented in chapter 4.

What Would You Do?

1. Suppose you have just begun working as an entry-level health promotion specialist in a midsized pharmaceutical firm. Your boss asks you to do a risk factor cost analysis to determine the most expensive risk factors in your workforce. She wants the analysis completed within a month to use in revising the current health promotion program. When you inquire about the availability of on-site medical claims data, your boss directs you to the benefits director who sheepishly informs you there is no data. You diplomatically inform the benefits director of the various benefits such data provide health management personnel and that you really need the data to complete your task in a timely manner. You then ask him to contact the off-site TPA to request aggregate claims and cost data reports over the past two years that distinguish employees from dependents and inpatient patterns from outpatient. He makes the request and is told by the TPA that these reports will cost $5,000 because they are not considered to be standard. The benefits director informs you that his budget is tight and that he cannot afford to pay the $5,000 report preparation fee. You really want to do the cost analysis and feel the only way to get the process underway is to get your boss and the benefits director to share responsibility for the $5,000 fee. What would you say to your boss and to the benefits director to persuade them to do this?

2. Suppose you have been asked to participate in your organization's cost management committee. In the first meeting, the committee chairperson shares examples of on-site data and the major goals. One of the goals is to identify the most expensive risk factors and determine appropriate risk-reduction interventions that will be implemented in the next 12-18 months. As director of your organization's health promotion programs, you volunteer to assist in conducting a risk factor cost appraisal. You explain that such an appraisal requires inpatient and outpatient claims data by DRG and ICD codes. You notice that the current on-site data is not separated by inpatient versus outpatient claims and is formatted only by MDC. Several committee members inquire as to why the separated data are required and in the course of replying, you begin to describe the value of risk factor weights. At this point, you see a lot of puzzled looks on the faces of committee members. How will you explain risk factor weights clearly to those on the committee with no background in WHP evaluation?

4

Financial Analysis

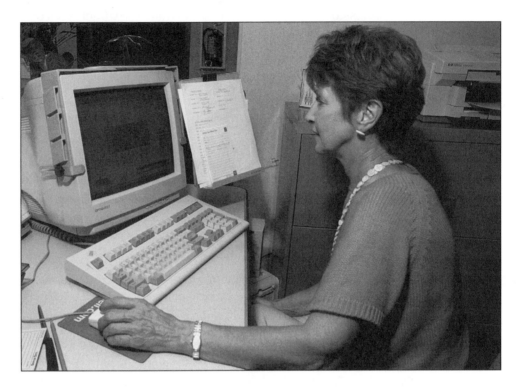

After reading this chapter and answering the questions at the end, you should be able to do the following:

- Distinguish between a non-econometric versus an econometric evaluation framework.

- Identify appropriate times to use a specific econometric tool.

- Project future benefits and costs of a particular intervention.

- Construct a sample forecasting framework.

- Distinguish between fixed versus variable costs.

- Identify and compare program costs against program benefits.

- Determine if an intervention is likely to pay for itself.

- Predict when a program is likely to pay for itself.

- Compare two or more interventions at the same time for cost-effectiveness.

The analysis tools in this chapter are all concerned only with the economic benefits and costs of a program. I present them based on the assumption that to intelligently evaluate any program, you must at the very least understand how much money it will cost and how much money it will save. Do not think, however, that quantification should be the sole basis for evaluation. Just because some factors cannot be measured does not mean they should be ignored. How, for example, can you quantify the pain and suffering of severe back pain or chronic depression? Although you can calculate the direct costs of treating a heart attack victim or discount a person's future job earnings lost from a disability, such noble benefits as human lives saved, preventing heart attacks, or easing chronic back pain are not easily translated into a financial benefit. Imagine the technical and ethical implications of trying to do so! Thus, although health promotion evaluation cannot be done apart from the objective facts that properly used econometric analysis tools can provide, neither should the subjectivity introduced by one's own values be avoided.

The tools covered in this chapter are forecasting, break-even analysis, cost-effectiveness analysis, and benefit-cost analysis. Once you have mastered each of these tools, you will be well equipped to help organizations answer their financial questions about their worksite health promotion programs.

Benefit/Cost Terminology

You will find many benefit/cost terms in this chapter. You will need to be familiar with the following benefit/cost terms to understand the material that follows.

Benefits

Benefit: a measurable entity that reflects an improved outcome such as health status, risk reduction, enhanced productivity, less absenteeism, higher profits, less expenses, and so on.

Direct benefit: a positive outcome relevant to the stated goals of an intervention.

Indirect benefit: a positive outcome that occurred in addition to a direct benefit, usually not relevant to the stated goals of an intervention, also called **opportunity benefit**.

Cost-avoidance benefit: what one is doing in creating indirect benefits because an indirect benefit is the amount of future dollars not spent rather than dollars actually saved and deposited.

Benefit variable: a benefit when it is used as a variable, also called **tangible benefit**.

Costs

Direct cost: an expected cost incurred to pay for essential items such as staff, medical costs, and so on.

Indirect cost: a cost that was unexpected or excessively higher than an expected cost.

Variable cost: a cost that fluctuates on a daily, monthly, quarterly, seasonal, or annual basis with the resources or the quantity (of products or services) sold that are used to implement an intervention. Usually, variable costs are calculated on a per-unit basis such as hourly labor, supplies, utilities, telephone expenses, and so forth. Variable costs are often influenced by external forces and thus are usually unpredictable.

Fixed cost: a cost that remains constant over time. Fixed costs are not affected by the quantity sold or paid resources. Examples include salaried personnel, rent, and insurance. They are rarely influenced by external forces and are thus predictable.

(continued)

Mixed costs: cost items that possess characteristics of both variable and fixed costs. Salaries, for example, could be a mixed cost if an hourly wage earner was promoted to a salaried position with a raise or if a salary earner was promoted and given a raise. Since none of the evaluation formulas can account for mixed costs, it is essential for every mixed cost to be defined as either fixed or variable. Each such cost will be treated as a variable cost or a fixed cost depending on the circumstances.

Operational costs: all the costs incurred in providing and sustaining a program intervention, usually considered to be all the direct costs of a program.

Opportunity cost: an undesirable and unexpected cost that interferes with the ability of an intervention to produce direct and indirect benefits.

Forecasting

Those who do not understand history are likely to repeat it. That saying is just as applicable to worksite health promotion efforts as it is to any other context. While no one knows what the future holds, decision makers who understand the past and how it influences the present are more likely to recognize and take advantage of opportunities in the future than those who do not appreciate the past. They are also more likely to foresee potential pitfalls and to avoid them. Using analyzed data, forecasting gauges how current trends may influence the future. According to Webster's Dictionary, to forecast means *to calculate or predict (some future event or condition) usually as a result of rational study and analysis of available pertinent data.*

Forecasting is an imperfect science. It must be approached with objectivity and realistic expectations, and it must be performed using accurate data and market-driven indexes (units of measurement that indicate change). The **consumer price index,** for example, indicates the rate of general inflation in the economy. In addition, forecasts should always take into account any demographic, social, financial, political, occupational, and technological changes or factors that could affect an organization and its employees. For instance, if you want to forecast on-the-job injuries, it is important to take into account the aging of a workforce and the availability of ergonomically enhanced equipment.

Although there are various ways to prepare a forecast, here is one reasonable sequence for doing key procedures:

1. Select a variable that can be measured.
2. Identify influential factors and select (or create) indexes that influence the variable.
3. Establish an appropriate time frame.
4. Create a customized forecast data table.
5. Obtain accurate and relevant data for indexes and an index baseline.
6. Compute a representative forecast baseline and prepare a customized forecast table.
7. Perform the calculations and record the results in a customized forecast table.

In the following section, we discuss the steps for preparing forecasts with each step being illustrated for both simple and complex forecasts. The difference between simple and complex forecasts becomes clearer in step two.

Step One: Select a Variable That Can Be Measured

What types of outcome variables can be forecasted? Virtually any variable is suitable for a forecast if it can be tracked over time with appropriate indexes. Outcomes that are particularly suitable for forecasting include the following:

- Health care utilization
- Health care expenses
- Accidents and injuries
- Program participation
- Migration into/out of health plans
- Turnover patterns
- Use of fitness facilities

Some variables can be viewed in different ways and therefore are subjected to different modes of measurement. Productivity, for example, could be measured in the following terms:

- Production/manufacturing—number of gadgets produced per day
- Qualitative—number of defects per 100,000 units produced
- Efficiency—number of people needed to properly operate a division

Be sure, when you are selecting your variable, that you think about whether it can be measured in more than one way and if so, make sure that you are measuring it in a way that will answer whatever questions management is asking.

Sample Forecasts

WHP planners need to be able to distinguish situations that call for either a simple forecast or a complex forecast. How to select variables in both cases is illustrated in the following sections.

Selecting a Variable for a Simple Forecast

Suppose that health management personnel in a midsize company of 500 employees select low back injury costs as the forecast variable. The variable was chosen because on-the-job back injuries had increased to an all-time high in the past six months. This variable is popular in many worksites because of its growing prevalence, its negative impact on productivity, and the significant amount of medical care dollars spent on it.

Selecting a Variable for a Complex Forecast

Suppose that health management personnel in a midsize company of 500 employees select health-related productivity loss as the forecast variable. The main reason for its selection was to gauge future health-related productivity costs if WHP program participation levels did not increase. Consequently, they establish an operational definition of lost productivity as *Direct and indirect costs borne by the employer for days lost that are attributed to health-related absences and disability.*

Step Two: Identify Influential Factors and Select (or Create) Indexes That Influence the Variable

Once you have selected the outcome variable you wish to forecast, you must identify the factors that influence it, then select or create indexes that will measure the rates of change in those factors as accurately as possible. In simple forecasts, the influential factors are for the most part no different from those that have affected standardized indexes. Customized indexes do not need to be created to track them; standardized indexes will adequately do the job. In complex forecasts, some of the influential factors are different from those that have affected standardized indexes; otherwise, they have changed at a different rate from those that have influenced standardized indexes. This factor makes it necessary for the evaluator to create customized indexes to complete the forecasts. Therefore, the distinction made clear in the following sample forecasts is that simple forecasts generally use only standardized indexes that account for no more than a few influential factors; complex forecasts generally combine both standardized and created indexes to account for the influential factors. Rarely will complex forecasts use only created indexes.

Determine Influential Factors

Once an outcome (dependent) variable has been selected for a forecast, it is necessary to identify its direct influences—that is, what influenced it in the past, what is currently influencing it, and anything that is expected to influence it during the time covered by your forecast. For example, virtually all businesses are concerned about rising health care costs and want to improve their cost-management efforts. Considering the inevitable year-to-year inflationary trend of these costs, employers need to identify past, present, and future factors that influence health care costs. Here are some general guidelines to help you decide when to consider each of the factors:

1. Incorporate present and past influential factors into your forecast only if you expect them to continue into the future.

2. If an influential factor has not been a factor in the past, there is no way of calculating or finding an index for it because the indexes have to be based on past rates of change. Therefore, it can't be used.

3. If a factor has not been historically influential in one's organization but has been in other organizations—and the WHP team predicts that it will soon be influential—that factor could still be used if standardized indexes or data from other companies were available to use.

The following is a partial listing of such factors. The *Future* column lists factors likely to influence corporate health care costs in the future. Those factors that currently influence costs and those that have influenced them are in the *Present* and *Past* columns, respectively.

Past	Present	Future
Medical inflation	Medical inflation	Medical inflation
Technology	Technology	Technology
Cost-shifting	Cost-shifting	Cost-shifting
Shadow pricing	Medicare	Medicare
Legislation	Legislation	Legislation
Varying standards	Varying standards	Varying standards
Workforce size	Workforce size	Workforce size
	Aging population	Aging population
	Sentinel effect	Limited discount options
		Internet purchasing

Begin by listing influential factors based on your knowledge, then explore the professional literature and solicit input from your health management colleagues.

Some of the periodicals that are reliable sources of the latest thinking in the field on this subject include

- *American Journal of Health Promotion,*
- *AWHP's Worksite Health,*
- *Business & Health,*
- *Employee Benefit Plan Review,*
- *Healthcare Informatics,* and
- *Journal of Occupational & Environmental Medicine.*

Illustrating Rates of Change: Nominal Versus Percentage Graphs

The values of virtually all the variables you can forecast change over time. When you are reviewing changes, it is important to know that the rate of nominal change may have a slope that appears to be quite different from the percentage of change in the same factor during the same time. This difference results from the fact that nominal values such as health care claims and costs vary within a significantly larger scale (per thousands of claims, per millions of dollars of costs) than the mere 100 points that define percentages. Figure 4.1 illustrates how the slope representing the nominal value (number of dollars) can look quite different from the slope representing the percentage of change by year, especially from 1996 to 1998. However, if you look closely, you will see that the directions of change do, in fact, coincide with each other. This distinction is important because graphs that consist of percentage changes can be visually misleading to observers since they often show different trend lines than those illustrated in a nominal graph. For example, nominal costs highlighted in figure 4.1 clearly show increased levels at each year despite the fact that the percentage change increase of 5% from 1996 to 1997 was actually lower than the previous year. Thus, decision makers should not rely exclusively on percentage changes for an accurate indication of actual changes.

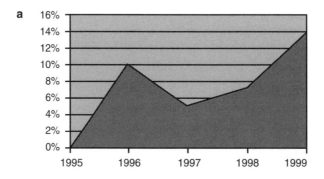

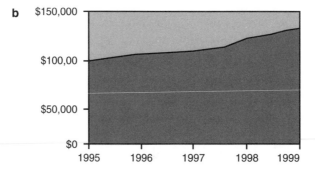

Figure 4.1 A comparison of *(a)* percentage changes versus *(b)* nominal changes over five years.

Select Standardized or Customized Indexes

In order to forecast future costs, you can assume that they will increase, but the question is, at what rate? Which indexes should be used to project future costs? At this point, the factors that influence health care come into play. Having determined every possible factor that may influence the variable you are forecasting, you must decide which, if any, of these factors you need to forecast, then you find or create indexes for each of those factors. For example, if you are forecasting health care costs to your employer, you may decide that it is sufficient to forecast the variable as a whole without distinguishing factors that may influence it. That is, rather than forecasting the cost of medical technology, the cost of insurance to the employer, and the aging population of your workforce—all influential factors—you may decide that using standardized indexes that have been influenced by all these factors will be precise enough, such as the retail and wholesale medical inflation indexes discussed next. On the other hand, you may decide that some of the factors influencing your company's bottom line for health care have an abnormally strong effect, so you need to take them into account more precisely. In this case, you need to treat each of them separately.

An organization wishing to forecast its health care costs may decide to use a standardized index that encompasses the changes in the variable as a whole because of the following reasons:

- It may not be aware of the various factors that drive corporate health care costs.
- It may be aware of the various factors that drive corporate health care costs but does not know how each of the factors independently influence these costs.
- It may believe that each of the factors that drive corporate health care costs have a similar influence; thus, there is no need to measure the independent influence of any single factor.

In contrast, another organization may be aware of certain factors that it believes could be disproportionately higher than the norm. Thus, the organization selects the following indexes for the reasons given:

- Pharmaceutical drug costs. The percentage of the company's total health care costs due to pharmaceutical costs has increased from 10% to 20% in the past two years.
- Medical technology. The company's health benefits plan has been expanded to include experimental treatments for cancer-related conditions. Health care economists expect such changes will increase corporate health care costs approximately 5%.
- Cost-shifting: Local hospital officials recently announced that the percentage of unpaid invoices has risen 10% in the past year.

If you are using standardized indexes, which ones should you use? If you are creating customized indexes, how do you know which ones to create? First, let's look at standardized indexes.

Selecting Standardized Indexes

If you decide to use standardized indexes, it is important to choose them carefully. If, for example, a company uses only the **consumer price index (CPI),** which is an indicator of general inflation rather than medical care inflation, to forecast its future health care costs, their forecasts will always be lower than actual health care expenses. Would it be sufficient then to depend on, say, the retail medical inflation rate to project future costs? It does indeed seem reasonable to use this tool to forecast year-to-year cost increases over the next several years. However, this single index does not provide forecasters with a range of **best case**, **worst case**, and **typical case** projections. Therefore, it is important to use several inflationary indexes to provide a full-scale forecast. Standardized indexes to consider in projecting health care inflation include the following:

- Retail medical inflation—the rate that small and midsize organizations typically pay for employee health care benefits
- Wholesale medical inflation—the rate (lower than retail) that larger organizations typically pay for health care
- Regional medical inflation—the composite, or average, rate of a region (e.g., the Southeast, the Midwest)
- Industry norm—the average rate that companies within a specific industry pay for employee health care benefits

Specific indexes are available from various government agencies such as the Health Care Financing Administration and Bureau of Labor Statistics, and major benefits consulting firms such as Milliman and Robertson, William Mercer, and Watson Wyatt.

Selecting Customized Indexes

Indexes specific to the company can be created by measuring the rate of change over a specified time frame. The following are examples of outcome variables and the factors that would influence them—each of which would need an index created:

- Outcome Variable: Fitness Center Participation
  - Percentage increase or decrease in the past 12 months
  - Percentage change in size of workforce expected in the next 12 months
  - Percentage change in employee age groups 20-29, 30-39, and so on
  - Percentage of employees expected to participate if new or expanded incentives are offered
- Outcome Variable: Injuries/Accidents
  - Percentage change in past year for specific types of injuries (e.g., sprains, carpal tunnel syndrome)
  - Percentage change in employees with occupations that experienced the greatest portion of injuries in the past year
- Outcome Variable: Risk Factor Incidence
  - Percentage change in total workforce (percent of employees expected to incur a risk factor) expected in the next 12 months
  - Percentage change in age groups currently with highest risk factor rates expected in the next 12 months
- Outcome Variable: Equipment Replacement Costs
  - Usage patterns (under- versus overuse compared to current level)
  - Multiply purchase price by the average annual inflation rate applicable to the specific type of equipment

Influential Factors and Indexes in Sample Forecasts

How to select influential factors and the indexes to forecast them is illustrated in the upcoming sections. In this step, the distinction between simple and complex forecasts becomes clearer. Note that in the simple forecast, only standardized indexes are used, and no unique influential factors are tracked; in the complex forecast, several influential factors are identified and custom indexes are created to track many of them.

The Simple Forecast

Because she had recently investigated her own company's rate of medical care inflation for other forecasts, the WHP specialist knew it was 9.5%, which fell between the standardized indexes for the wholesale medical inflation rate and the retail medical inflation rate. Thus, she suspected that there was no unusual influential factor on low back costs in their workforce. To be certain this was a valid conclusion, she studied in-house records on low back injuries. Again she found no unusual increase in low back injury incidence or any other factors that seemed any different from those of the general population. Thus, she decided that standardized indexes—indicating rates of change in medical care cost inflation plus the company's medical care inflation rate, which she already knew—would be adequate for forecasting best to worst case scenarios for her company's future back care costs, assuming no intervention or program was instituted to improve the rate of back injury. Moreover, she was quite sure that even the best case scenario (one created without factoring the specifics of their workforce, such as its rising average age) would show very significant increases in the cost of low back injuries in the next few years. She believed, in fact, that they would be so high that management would be persuaded of the value of instituting back care programs even without the time-consuming procedures required by a complex forecast. Thus, the specialist decided to begin with a simple forecast, reasoning that if the numbers did not seem particularly persuasive, she could then go back and do the more precise calculations necessary for a complex forecast. The specific indexes that she selected were the wholesale medical inflation, retail medical inflation, her company's medical care inflation, and consumer price inflation.

The Complex Forecast

After doing a review of the professional literature and conducting an in-house culture audit, the health management team believed the following factors were primarily responsible for the increase in the company's health-related lost productivity:

- Liberal **sick leave** policy
- High level of work dissatisfaction among employees
- Lack of incentives for good work attendance
- No on-site employee health promotion and risk-reduction programs
- Increased prevalence of modifiable risk factors and their associated costs

Among the preceding factors, suppose that only the second and last had previously been tracked at the worksite. The remaining factors had never been monitored; thus, they could not have quantified indexes created for them for use in a forecast. Evaluators were then limited to using at most only two factors, and they now had to determine if both were applicable to the forecast. In making this decision, they struggled with the prospect that they could end up with only one quantifiable index in the forecast, which might reduce its degree of objectivity. After some debate, they decided to use the prevalence and cost of selected modifiable risk factors as the sole factor among the original five. They reasoned that they would be tracking multiple risk factors and would by necessity be using a separate index to forecast each; therefore, they would be reintroducing some measure of objectivity into their forecast. They chose as risk factors physical inactivity, obesity, hypertension, and diabetes. They decided to create two indexes per risk factor:

- The average percentage increase in prevalence of each risk factor over the last four years
- The average percentage increase in the cost to the company for days lost due to each risk factor in the past four years.

The steps they followed to determine the rates of change in each of these eight indexes (two indexes for each of four risk factors) are discussed in detail on pages 92-94.

Step Three: Establish an Appropriate Time Frame

Now it is appropriate to establish the chronological framework of your forecast. The time frame should take into account that a forecast may be extremely vulnerable to daily and weekly events and thus may lose some validity (accuracy) over a longer time frame. For example, general inflation (consumer price index) and medical inflation both experienced an up-and-down **roller-coaster** phenomenon throughout the 1990s.

Two guidelines frequently used to determine how long a forecasting time frame should be are as follows:

- If the forecast variable showed little or no year-to-year change in the past four to five years, it is relatively safe to use a similar time frame for the forecast.
- If the variable to be forecasted showed substantial year-to-year change over the past few years, it is appropriate to either limit the forecast to a shorter time frame (one to two years, for example) or use a multiyear average to calculate the forecast. For example, the average annual return of the S&P 500 Stock Index for the period of 1994-1998 was 22.4%; yet, there was wide year-to-year volatility— even in consecutive years—as evidenced by a low of 1% in 1994 to a high of 38% in the following year.

Establishing a Time Frame in the Sample Forecasts

We now discuss how to establish a time frame. What follows is an illustration for both the simple and complex sample forecasts.

The Simple Forecast

All the indexes used in the forecast were monitored on a year-to-year basis. Therefore, a time frame of several 12-month intervals was selected for the forecast.

The Complex Forecast

The selected risk factors (physical inactivity, obesity, hypertension, and diabetes) had been monitored annually for the past five years via health screenings and a health risk appraisal. However, risk factor cost data had only been identified over the past year through a PRFCA conducted as part of a recent claims data analysis. Since risk factor costs had been tracked over a period of 12 months, health management personnel decided that the forecast should contain several 12-month intervals.

Step Four: Create a Customized Forecast Data Table

You can establish the **blueprint** of your forecast once all the influential factors have been identified, the appropriate indexes have been selected, and a time frame has been established. This blueprint is nothing more than a blank table into which you can plug the results of your calculations. It will serve as a framework to keep you focused on the elements that you need to take into account as you perform your forecast. In preparing such a framework, make sure you incorporate all of the elements shown in figure 4.2 and label the time frame columns according to the chronological framework you have established for the forecast:

- Outcome variable—the dependent variable that is influenced by one or more indexes. You will need a separate table for each outcome variable.
- Forecast indexes—specific indexes you will use to project how the outcome variable will change over the specified time frame. Record the names of the indexes as well as the percentages they indicate in the first column.
- Baseline—the current value of the outcome variable. Record these in the second column.
- Time frame—the periods of time you are planning to forecast. Write these in the remaining columns. Include as many columns as necessary for your time frame.
- Quantitative data—numbers that reflect the predicted quantitative changes throughout the designated time frame. Once you have made your calculations, record these figures in the appropriate time frame columns.

Outcome variable:				
Forecast index		Baseline	Year	Year
	(%)			
	(%)			
	(%)			
	(%)			
	(%)			

Figure 4.2 Basic table for recording forecast data. Complex forecasts that use influential factors for the indexes, rather than several indexes that track the same variable, will add a *Totals* row (see next page).

If the outcome variable will be forecast as a whole, the number of rows will correspond to the number of indexes you are using for the forecast. If you break the outcome variable down into several factors defined by the influential factors, you may need to add a row for the total. The sample complex forecast illustrates the use of the *Totals* row.

Creating a Table for Recording Forecast Data for Sample Forecasts

Creating data recording tables is illustrated in the following sections. Both simple and complex sample forecasts are included in the discussion.

The Simple Forecast

The company WHP specialist created a customized table for recording data. It included all four of the indexes she had chosen and also a time frame (see figure 4.3).

The Complex Forecast

A customized forecast table was created to record the baseline and the forecasted annual changes for the cost of each risk factor in terms of lost productivity. The version

Outcome variable: Cost of low back injuries				
Forecast index	Baseline	Year 1	Year 2	Year 3
Wholesale medical inflation @ 7%	$			
Retail medical inflation @ 10%	$			
Company's medical care inflation @ 9.5%	$			
Consumer price index @ 1.5%	$			

Figure 4.3   Customized table in which data for simple forecast will be recorded.

Outcome variable: Health-related lost productivity				
Forecast index	Baseline	Year 1	Year 2	Year 3
Physical inactivity risk factor (rf) prevalence (%)				
Cost to company for days lost to physical inactivity (%)				
Obesity rf prevalence (%)				
Cost to company for days lost to obesity (%)				
Hypertension rf prevalence (%)				
Cost to company for days lost to hypertension (%)				
Diabetes rf prevalence (%)				
Cost to company for days lost to diabetes (%)				
Totals				

Figure 4.4   Customized table in which data for complex forecast will be recorded.

of the table shown in figure 4.4 contains only the names of the selected indexes and the time frame. For each index, the forecasters have yet to establish the rates of change, the baseline, and, of course, the annual changes that can be predicted based on the indexes' rates of change and baselines.

Step Five: Obtain Accurate and Relevant Data for Indexes and an Index Baseline

After selecting a variable to forecast, you need to assess your data resources. Use only the most recent and credible data to establish baselines and to select standardized forecasts or create customized ones. This will ensure that your forecasts are characterized by the following traits:

- Precise: They feature as small a margin of error as possible.
- Appropriate: They are relevant to a specific business, industry, group, or age distribution.
- Applicable: They are targeted to the situation being analyzed.
- Valuable: They provide decision makers with information that is useful for strategic planning.

Review *Working With Data* (pages 33-45) to remind yourself of how to ensure that the data with which you work are valid.

The desirable features of a forecast made using recent and credible data may seem obvious. But evaluators do not always design their forecasts to be precise, appropriate, applicable, and valuable.

Many public and private sector research firms and professional associations provide data in various formats that can be used in preparing specific types of forecasts. The following is a list of organizations with the type of data that they can supply. Some of them may charge a fee, so you may want to inquire first.

Absenteeism	Bureau of National Affairs
	National Institute of Occupational Safety & Health
Accidents/injuries	American Red Cross
	Crawford and Company
	Occupational Safety and Health Administration
Health care utilization/costs	American Hospital Association
	Employee Benefits Research Institute
	Health Care Financing Administration
	Bureau of Labor Statistics
	Society of Actuaries
	Marion Merrill Dow
	Milliman and Robertson
	A. Foster Higgins
	Society of Prospective Medicine
	William Mercer, Inc.
Inflation rates	A. Foster Higgins
	Health Care Financing Administration
	Bureau of Labor Statistics
Participation rates	Association for Worksite Health Promotion
	American College of Sports Medicine
	International Health, Racquet and Sportsclub Association
Productivity	Bureau of Labor Statistics
	International Quality and Productivity Center
	William Mercer, Inc.
Risk factors	Centers for Disease Control and Prevention
	Behavioral Risk Factor Surveillance System (BRFSS)
	National Health and Nutrition Evaluation Survey (NHANES)
	Department of Health and Human Services (HHS)
Workers' compensation	National Council on Compensation Insurance
	Workers' Compensation Research Institute
	Crawford and Company

Creating Indexes for a Sample Complex Forecast

The easiest way to calculate indexes is

1. to create custom tables for recording data similar to the ones for recording the forecast data,
2. to fill in the data, and
3. to perform the calculations called for by the table.

This technique is illustrated for only the complex forecast as the simple forecast did not require the specialist to create any indexes.

Creating a Table for Calculating Custom Indexes

To generate the indexes that they needed to perform their forecast, the staff first created a customized index calculation table (see figure 4.5). Note the similarities to figure 4.2, such as the framework for the customized table for the forecasting data. Like figure 4.2, this customized table has a row for each index, and it has columns for the index names, the baseline, and the years of tracked data. There are differences, however:

- The index value is not recorded with the index name.
- A column for *% change* is added after each year's data.
- A column for *Index value*, which is the average of the *% change* columns, is added at the right side of the table.

Outcome variable: Health-related lost productivity

Forecast index	Baseline year	Year 2	% change between baseline and year 2	Year 3	% change between year 2 and year 3	Year 4	% change between year 3 and year 4	Index value
Physical inactivity rf prevalence								
Company's cost for days lost to physical inactivity								
Obesity rf prevalence								
Company's cost for days lost to obesity								
Hypertension rf prevalence								
Company's cost for days lost to hypertension								
Diabetes rf prevalence								
Company's cost for days lost to diabetes								

Figure 4.5 Customized index calculation table.

Obtaining Data and Calculating Indexes

After creating the table, the health management team obtained the data necessary for figuring the value of each index. In order to establish that value, it was necessary for the team to obtain data on

- the prevalence of each risk factor (physical inactivity, obesity, hypertension, and diabetes) for the past five years, and
- the cost to the company for each of those years of productivity lost due to each factor.

The figures for the prevalence of each risk factor were obtained from previous annual health risk appraisals, which in turn had been figured from employee's health records. The percentage of employees having each risk factor during the first year were placed in the risk factor prevalence rows in the *Baseline year* column, those for the second year in the *Year 2* column, and so on.

The annual cost to the company of lost productivity for each of the risk factors in the years tracked was obtained by a five-step process. Each listed step is illustrated by the figures obtained for year four for physical inactivity.

1. Ask the payroll department for the median salary of each year and the average number of employees in the company for that year:

   median salary = $48,000; average number of employees = 500

2. Ask the HR department for the average number of hours lost each year due to disability by each employee with the tracked risk factor:

   average number of hours lost each year due to physical inactivity: 11.6

3. Multiply the prevalence of each risk factor for each year by the average number of employees that year to calculate the total number of employees each year with the risk factor. For example, in year four, the prevalence of physical inactivity in the workforce was 60% (0.6 in decimal terms), and the size of the workforce was 500 workers:

   physical inactivity prevalence rate (0.6) $\times$ total number of workers (500) = 300 workers who are physically inactive.

4. Divide the average number of hours lost each year by the total hours in the work year (2000) to arrive at the average percentage of hours lost that year by workers with the tracked risk factor:

   average hours lost (11.6) divided by total hours in the work year (2000) = .0058

5. Multiply the number of employees each year with the risk factor by the average percent of hours lost due to the risk factor, by the median salary for that year:

   number of employees with risk factor (300) $\times$ average % hours lost due to risk factor (.0058) $\times$ median salary ($48,000) = $83,520

This final figure was placed in the space for *Company's cost for days lost to physical inactivity* in the *Year 4* column of the customized index calculation table.

A more detailed explanation of a similar five-step process is presented in step 6 of the forecast (pages 94-97). If you have questions remaining about the steps, they will be answered in that section.

Forecast index	Baseline year	Year 2	% change between baseline year and year 2	Year 3	% change between year 2 and year 3	Year 4	% change between year 3 and year 4	Index value
Physical inactivity rf prevalence	57.3%	58.9%		59.5%		60%		
Company's cost for days lost to physical inactivity	$73,346	$76,963		$81,014		$83,520		

Figure 4.6   Customized index data obtained and listed for each year.

Forecast index	Baseline year	Year 2	% change between baseline year and year 2	Year 3	% change between year 2 and year 3	Year 4	% change between year 3 and year 4	Index value
Physical inactivity rf prevalence	57.3%	58.9%	**2.79%**	59.5%	**1%**	60%	**.08%**	**1.29%**
Company's cost for days lost to physical inactivity	$73,346	$76,963	**4.9%**	$81,014	**5.2%**	$83,520	**3%**	**4.36%**

Figure 4.7   Customized index data with annual percentage changes and the four-year average index vlaue.

At this point, the team had recorded the data for risk factor prevalence and the answers to the five-step process of calculating the company's cost for lost productivity for each risk factor for each year in the appropriate columns in their chart. (Figure 4.6 shows these figures recorded in the first two rows.) Next, they had to calculate the percentage of change between each two years.

Finally, the team averaged the percentage of change between each two years (2.79%, 1%, and .08%) to arrive at the index rate (1.29%), which they recorded in the last column, *Index value*. Figure 4.7 shows in bold the figures they calculated and recorded in the first two rows of this step.

Figure 4.8 shows the entire customized index calculation table for the complex forecast. The data for the baseline year and the three years after it have been entered in the appropriate columns. The results of the calculations for the percentage of change between each two years have been entered in the appropriate *% change* columns. The averages of the percentage of change between each two years have been inserted in the *Index value* column.

Once they had the value of each index, they inserted it after the appropriate index name in their customized data recording chart. Figure 4.9 shows the appropriate section of the forecast data recording chart with the index values filled in.

Step Six: Compute a Representative Forecast Baseline and Prepare a Customized Forecast Table

If you're going to forecast anything, of course, you must know the point from which you are starting. This is the baseline for your forecast.

Outcome variable: Health-related lost productivity

Forecast index	Baseline year	Year 2	% change between baseline year and year 2	Year 3	% change between year 2 and year 3	Year 4	% change between year 3 and year 4	Index value
Physical inactivity rf prevalence	57.3%	58.9%	2.79%	59.5%	1%	60%	.08%	1.29%
Company's cost for days lost to physical inactivity	$73,346	$76,963	4.9%	$81,014	5.2%	$83,520	3%	4.36%
Obesity rf prevalence	38.2%	38.8%	1.5%	39.2%	1%	40%	2%	1.5%
Company's cost for days lost to obesity	$69,264	$74,638	7.7%	$80,256	7.5%	$84,480	5.2%	6.8%
Hypertension rf prevalence	19.25%	19.4%	.07%	19.8%	2%	20%	1%	1.02%
Company's cost for days lost to hypertension	$56,428	$61,603	9.1%	$66,960	8.6%	$72,000	7.5%	8.4%
Diabetes rf prevalence	4.85%	4.87%	.04%	4.95%	16%	5%	1%	.4%
Company's cost for days lost to diabetes	$29,487	$31,186	5.7%	$32,486	4.1%	$34,560	6.3%	5.36%

Figure 4.8 The entire customized index calculation table for the complex forecast.

Forecast index
Physical inactivity rf prevalence (+1.29%)
Cost to company for days lost to physical inactivity (+4.36%)
Obesity rf prevalence (+1.5%)
Cost to company for days lost to obesity (+6.8%)
Hypertension rf prevalence (+1.02%)
Cost to company for days lost to hypertension (8.4%)
Diabetes rf prevalence (+.4%)
Cost to company for days lost to diabetes (5.36%)
Total—risk factor (rf) _____
Total—costs _____

Figure 4.9 A section of the forecast data recording chart with index values filled in.

Say, for example, that you are forecasting the likely costs of a low back injury reduction program. First, you need to review low back injuries and costs over the past several years to develop a good baseline. When you have several years of retrospective data on low back injuries that consistently show

- a year-to-year downward trend,
- no year-to-year change, or
- a year-to-year upward trend,

it is acceptable to use the last year's performance as the baseline. See table 4.1 for three sets of data listing the number of low back injuries at different worksites for the past four years.

Table 4.1   Data Sets Showing Different Trends

	Upward trend	No change trend	Downward trend
4 years ago	17	17	17
3 years ago	19	18	15
2 years ago	23	17	13
1 year ago	28	18	11

One shows a clear upward trend; one shows no significant change, and one shows a clear downward trend.

The data, however, are not usually so clear. It is common to see year-to-year data mimicking a roller coaster—going up and down in a chaotic order. If that is the case, it is important to establish a baseline that does not favor the best or worst end of a multiyear trend, but rather one that reflects a middle-of-the-road point. For example, consider figure 4.10, which illustrates significant quarter-to-quarter changes in an organization's absenteeism in the past two years.

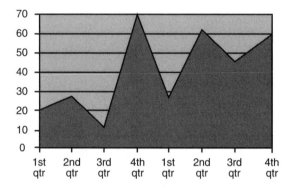

Figure 4.10   Quarterly absenteeism in days per 1,000 employees for two consecutive years.

There are various ways to buffer the volatility shown in figure 4.10 and thus enhance the odds of computing a representative baseline:

• The first technique is to compute the mathematical **median** (midpoint). The median is probably most familiar to you as the **50th percentile**. The median is the value that exactly separates the upper half of the distribution from the lower half. Simply put, 50% of the scores are lower than the median and the other 50% are greater than the median. In order to compute the median, first list all scores in ranked order:

70   63   59   45   27   27   20   10

Since there is an even number of scores, select the two most centralized scores; add them (45 + 27) and divide the sum (72) by two (2) to compute the median: 72 divided by 2 = 36. Thus, the median appears as follows:

70   63   59   45   <u>36</u>   27   27   20   10

If you have an odd number of scores, the median score is simply the middle entry:

70   63   59   45   <u>45</u>   27   27   20   10

- Second, compute the **mode**. The French expression *a la mode* literally means *in vogue* or *in style,* which is exactly what the mode is—the score that is made most frequently, the one that is most *in style.* The mode is easily identified by visually scanning the scores. But because it is the crudest measure of central tendency, it is not used as often as either the median or mean. The mode in the following range of numbers is 27 since it appears twice:

$$70 \quad 63 \quad 59 \quad 45 \quad 27 \quad 27 \quad 20 \quad 10$$

You can see from this list that the most common score is not necessarily the most representative index to use.

- Third, compute the arithmetic mean. The **mean** is more commonly known as the average. The mean can be easily computed by adding up all the scores and dividing by the number of scores, as follows:

$$70 + 63 + 59 + 45 + 27 + 27 + 20 + 10 = 321.$$

There are eight (8) scores, so, 321 divided by 8 = 40.125, which is the mean.

Because there is such a wide difference between the highest and lowest scores in this series, the mean of 40.125 may not be a good index to use as a baseline. In certain situations, the series may become more representative of the central tendency if we drop the highest and lowest scores (the **outliers**). In this case, however, when we drop the outliers (70 and 10), we compute a mean quite similar to the previous mean of 40.125:

$$63 + 59 + 45 + 27 + 27 + 20 = 241, \text{ divided by } 6 = 40.166.$$

The similar means are due, in large part, to the close proximity between the highest score (70) and the second and third highest scores (63, 59). Thus, in this instance, the elimination of outliers was not necessary to compute a representative baseline. Eliminating outliers is most appropriate when there is a wide disparity between the scores at either the higher or the lower end.

- Fourth, calculate the sum of the highest and lowest scores only, then divide by two (2) to calculate an average. With the same series of numbers, then, the results would be 70 + 10 = 80, which would be divided by two (2), to yield an average of 40.

- Finally, you could use data only from the most recent year.

If a measure of central tendency is a single value that best represents the performance of the group as a whole, which single value should be used? If, using the same set of scores, you compute the mean (with and without outliers), the median, the mode, and the highest and lowest scores divided by two, very rarely will all answers be identical. Which one then will give us the **best single value** that describes the entire distribution? What are the advantages and disadvantages of each option?

First of all, we should ignore the mode since it is a rather crude measure of central tendency. The mean is most often given as a measure of central tendency. This option provides you with a multiyear perspective and historical trending, but it gives equal representation to each year; therefore, it may not properly reflect the current situation. Eliminating outliers when you calculate the mean keeps them from disproportionately influencing the norm, yet it may not reveal the full range of year-to-year changes. If you calculate the mean using only the highest and lowest scores, you fully account for the best case and worst case scenarios, yet you may lose the influence of the most typical scores. Using the data only from the most recent year may reflect the current situation most clearly, but it does not account for any year-to-year changes or trends.

There are many instances where the median is a valuable statistic. It is not affected by extreme or atypical values as much as the mean is, so it is very useful in situations where the distribution is either positively or negatively skewed. For example, suppose the majority of employees reported on a health assessment questionnaire that they were experiencing high levels of on-the-job stress. Since the distribution would show a strong skewness on the high stress side of the continuum, the median would factor in the low and moderate stress scores while the average (mean) score would be inflated because of the disproportionately high percentage of highly stressed people.

In addition to considering the advantages and disadvantages of each option, you should take other factors in your situation into account as you decide how to use the data:

- Amount of retrospective data available. If several periods of data are available, evaluators usually consider all data and select one of the four preceding options based on the direction of the year-to-year changes.

- Degree of change in data. If there is a significant upward or downward trend over several intervals of data, evaluators tend to use an average of the two most recent intervals.

- Perceived validity (accuracy) of data. If evaluators suspect that data in one or more of the intervals are questionable in content or its source, they will usually either eliminate the suspicious data from consideration or give it less weight than other data.

- Consistency (reliability) of data. If data are similar over several time intervals, evaluators tend to select the most recent score or compute a multiyear average as the baseline. In contrast, if data exhibit a consistent trend (upward, downward, or stable) for all time intervals except the most recent, evaluators tend to give equal if not more credit to the trend than to the most recent score.

- Philosophy and goals of evaluation. If the climate calls for a conservative approach to evaluation, evaluators tend to use **worst case** data for the baseline to minimize unintentional stacking of the deck.

If, after considering all the factors discussed above, you still have difficulty deciding on which approach to take, discuss the pros and cons of using a specific baseline approach with your peers or consult selected organizations or associations for national or industry-specific norms (see appendix, page 189).

Computing Baselines for the Sample Forecasts

How the baselines were established for both the simple and the complex sample forecasts is presented in the following sections. Note that the process for computing the baselines for the complex forecast is very similar to that described above for filling in the chart used to calculate indexes. This process is discussed in greater detail.

Establishing a Baseline for a Simple Forecast

Since each index for the simple forecast was used to predict the same thing (future annual costs to the company of low back claims), the baseline was the same for each. This was the company's annual medical cost for low back injuries at the beginning of the period being forecasted. This figure was $50,000, and the WHP specialist recorded it in the customized data table for each index, as shown in figure 4.11.

Computing Baselines for a Complex Forecast

To establish a representative baseline for each of the influential factors in the complex forecast, evaluators were able to use in-house sources. The current prevalence of each

Forecast index	Baseline
Wholesale medical inflation @ 7%	**$50,000**
Retail medical inflation @ 10%	**$50,000**
Company's medical inflation @ 9.5%	**$50,000**
Consumer price index @ 1.5%	**$50,000**

Figure 4.11   First two columns of customized table for simple forecast filled in.

risk factor (physical inactivity, obesity, hypertension, and diabetes) was established by looking at the results of the company's most recent annual health risk appraisal. The average number of disability days per employee with the tracked risk factors was determined by examining records kept by the human resources office of the company. The results of this examination are recorded in table 4.2 with the number of workers with each risk factor recorded in the baseline column to establish prevalence.

Next, evaluators contacted the payroll department to obtain the monetary value of the median compensation (salary and benefits) per employee paid by the organization. The median compensation of $48,000 was applied to the total number of absent and disability days in computing the following lost productivity cost values, as shown in table 4.3.

As a result of the computation shown in table 4.3, a baseline cost to the company of days lost per selected risk factor was established and listed in the customized table for recording data for the complex forecast. This section of the table as filled out up to current step is shown in figure 4.12.

Computing a Baseline in the Absence of Company Data

What could the evaluators in the complex sample forecast have done if the company's records were not sufficient to supply them with the information they needed? They could have consulted other comparable worksites, conducted an Internet search for appropriate research articles, or contacted selected associations for data on how the

Table 4.2   Days Lost per Employee Due to Tracked Risk Factors

Risk factor	Risk factor % (#)	Disability days (hours)*
Physical inactivity	60% (300)	1.45 (11.6)
Obesity	40% (200)	2.2 (17.6)
Hypertension	20% (100)	3.75 (30.0)
Diabetes	5% (25)	7.2 (57.6)

*Averages

Table 4.3   Dollar Value of Productivity Lost Due to Risk Factors

Risk factor	# of at-risk employees	Lost hours % of work*	Median compensation	Cost of lost productivity
Physical inactivity	300 (60%)	.0058	$48,000	$83,520
Obesity	200 (40%)	.0088	$48,000	$84,480
Hypertension	100 (20%)	.015	$48,000	$72,000
Diabetes	25 (5%)	.0288	$48,000	$34,560

*Total hours lost divided by 2000 (based on 50 weeks @ 40 hours per week)

Forecast index	Baseline
Physical inactivity risk factor (rf) prevalence (+1.29%)	300
Cost to company of days lost to physical inactivity (+4.36%)	$83,520
Obesity rf prevalence (+1.5%)	200
Cost to company of days lost to obesity (+6.8%)	$84,480
Hypertension rf prevalence (+1.02%)	100
Cost to company of days lost to hypertension (8.4%)	$72,000
Diabetes rf prevalence (+.4%)	25
Cost to company of days lost to diabetes (5.36%)	$34,560

Figure 4.12 Index and baseline columns filled out in customized table for recording data for the complex forecast.

tracked risk factors have affected workforces comparable to their own. Having done so, they would have found that each resource used different methodological and analytical approaches. For example, one research study might have tracked working-age adults at several worksites while another could have used statistics on both worksites and the general community. Thus, it would be vital for evaluators to use only those data sources that worked with populations that matched those of their own company. Had they had such data available and had they carefully evaluated the sources, they could calculate composite averages for their influential factors with some confidence, knowing that the baselines would be reasonably close to their own statistics. Possible sources used in the computations include the following:

- Physical inactivity—American Heart Association; *Business & Health; Circulation: Journal of the American Heart Association; Journal of the American Medical Association; Journal of Occupational and Environmental Medicine; Medicine & Science in Sports & Exercise*

- Obesity—*Archives of Internal Medicine; Business & Health; Behavioral Medicine;* First Chicago Corporation; *Obesity Research*

- Hypertension—*American Journal of Hypertension; Business & Health;* Dietary Approaches to Stop Hypertension (DASH); National Heart, Lung and Blood Institute

- Diabetes—American Diabetes Association; *Business & Health; Diabetes; Public Health Reports*

Step Seven: Perform the Calculations and Record the Results

The final step is to perform the necessary calculations based on the information currently in each of your forecast tables. This information contains the names, the percentage rates, and your baselines for each of your selected or created indexes. The calculations based on these data will yield the figures necessary for filling in the remainder of the table.

Performing the Calculations on the Sample Forecasts

The clearest way to understand how to complete the forecast is to look at the samples we have been following throughout this section. They are presented in the next section.

Completing the Forecast Table and Performing the Calculations for a Simple Forecast

The WHP specialist has already established that the current cost to the company for medical care of low back injuries is $50,000. As seen in table 4.4, she used indexes for which the rates were already established. These are given again along with their relevance to low back claim costs.

Index	Inflation rate	Relevance to low back claim cost
Wholesale MI	7% (.07)	High
Retail MI	10% (.10)	High
Company	9.5% (.095)	Very high
CPI	1.5% (.015)	Moderate

Thus, to calculate the *Year 1* figure for each index, she first adds 1.00 to the decimal equivalent of the index. For example, for the Wholesale Medical Index, she would add 1.00 to .07, which would equal 1.07. She does this to preserve the value of the previous column. After doing so, she multiplies the baseline by this new figure. Using our example, she would multiply $50,000 by 1.07, which is $53,500. She would then put this figure in the first row under *Year 1*. To calculate *Year 2,* she would multiply the *Year 1* figure in the first row ($53,500) by 1.07, which would give her the answer $57,245. She would write this under *Year 2* in row one. To calculate *Year 3,* she would multiply the *Year 2* figure in row one by 1.07 to yield the answer $61,252. She would record this under *Year 3* in row one. She would then follow the same procedure for each row. Table 4.4 illustrates this process for each of the indexes.

When these calculations are performed and the answers recorded in the forecast table (figure 4.13), the forecast is complete. You can see that the forecasted low back claim cost ranges from approximately $52,000 (at CPI) to approximately $66,500 (at Retail Medical Inflation).

Completing the Forecast Table and Performing the Calculations for a Complex Forecast

The final procedure for the complex forecast was to subject each of the baselines in the forecast table to the designated annual percentage change for each year within the

Table 4.4   Calculations for Simple Forecast

Index	Baseline	Year 1	Year 2	Year 3
Wholesale MI	$50,000	× 1.07 = $53,500	× 1.07 = $57,245	× 1.07 = $61,252
Retail MI	$50,000	× 1.10 = $55,000	× 1.10 = $60,500	×1.10 = $66,550
Company	$50,000	× 1.095 = $54,750	× 1.095 = $59,951	× 1.095 = $65,646
CPI	$50,000	× 1.015 = $50,750	× 1.015 = $51,511	× 1.015 = $52,284

Forecast index	Baseline	Year 1	Year 2	Year 3
Wholesale medical inflation @ 7%	**$50,000**	$53,500	$57,245	$61,252
Retail medical inflation @ 10%	**$50,000**	$55,000	$60,500	$66,550
Company's medical care inflation @ 9.5%	**$50,000**	$54,750	$59,951	$65,646
Consumer price index @ 1.5%	**$50,000**	$50,750	$51,511	$52,284

Figure 4.13   Customized table in which data for simple forecast have been recorded.

forecasted time frame, just as it was done in the simple forecast. Table 4.5 illustrates the calculations performed for the complex forecast.

Having completed their calculations, the staff completed filling in the forecast table as illustrated in figure 4.14. They added up each column and could see that lost productivity costs tied to the selected risk factors were estimated to rise by over $59,000 by year 3.

Table 4.5 Calculations for Complex Forecast

Index	Baseline	Year 1	Year 2	Year 3
Physical inactivity risk factor prevalence (+1.29%)	300	× 1.0129 = 303.8	× 1.0129 = 307.7	× 1.0129 = 311.7
Company's cost for days lost to physical inactivity (+4.36%)	$83,520	× 1.0436 = $87,161	× 1.0436 = $90,961	× 1.0436 = $94,927
Obesity risk factor prevalence (+1.5%)	200	× 1.015 = 203	× 1.015 = 206	× 1.015 = 209
Company's cost for days lost to obesity (+6.8%)	$84,480	× 1.068 = $90,224	× 1.068 = $96,359	× 1.068 = $102,912
Hypertension risk factor prevalence (+1.02%)	100	× 1.0102 = 101.02	× 1.0102 = 102.05	× 1.0102 = 103.09
Company's cost for days lost to hypertension (+8.4%)	$72,000	× 1.084 = $78,048	× 1.084 = $84,604	× 1.084 = $91,710
Diabetes risk factor prevalence (+.4%)	25	× 1.004 = 25.1	× 1.004 = 25.2	× 1.004 = 25.3
Company's cost for days lost to diabetes (+5.36%)	$34,560	× 1.0536 = $36,412	× 1.0536 = $38,364	× 1.0536 = $44,420

Forecast index	Baseline	Year 1	Year 2	Year 3
Physical inactivity rf prevalence (+1.29%)	300	303	307	311
Cost to company for days lost to physical inactivity (+4.36%)	$83,520	$87,161	$90,961	$94,927
Obesity rf prevalence (+1.5%)	200	203	206	209
Cost to company for days lost to obesity (+6.8%)	$84,480	$90,224	$96,359	$102,912
Hypertension rf prevalence (+1.02%)	100	101	102	103
Cost to company for days lost to hypertension (8.4%)	$72,000	$78,048	$84,604	$91,710
Diabetes rf prevalence (+.4%)	25	25.1	25.2	25.3
Cost to company of days lost to diabetes (5.36%)	$34,560	$36,412	$38,364	$44,420
Total—risk factor	625	632	640	648
Total—costs	$274,560	$291,845	$310,288	$333,969

Figure 4.14 Customized table in which data for a complex forecast have been recorded.

Forecasting Potential Cost-Avoidance Benefits

One of the most common uses of forecasting is determining potential cost savings, also known as cost-avoidance benefits. For example, suppose an organization is currently spending $100,000 every six months on medical treatment for low back injuries. Upon reviewing retrospective claims data, we see that back injury costs have risen 10% each of the past five years. In its quest to stem these rising costs, the employer hires a local health promotion firm to design a low back injury prevention program. The firm will charge the employer $15,000 annually to design the program and monitor it semiannually. In doing so, the firm has promised the employer that the new program will meet the following goals:

- Make a positive impact within the initial six months of operation by raising morale, boosting communications, and generating teamwork.
- Contain low back injury claim costs at 50% of the nonintervention rate (5% versus 10%).
- Produce cost-avoidance savings that will offset programming and medical care costs within 12 months.

To check out the economics, you could use forecasting to compare projected low back injury and program intervention costs against low back injury costs with the program versus without the program.

The projected costs of the two options are shown in table 4.6. You can see that if the company does hire the health promotion firm and they perform as promised, the organization would have saved or avoided spending nearly $50,000 by the four-year mark.

Forecasting techniques provide decision makers with information to gauge possible scenarios in the future. Since forecasts can be vulnerable to the volatility of a changing economy, many forecasters prefer to incorporate a range of conservative-to-liberal indexes in their prognostications. With such a broad-based vision, decision makers are more likely to make well-informed planning and budgeting decisions than if they have forecasts based on only one index.

Table 4.6 A Comparison of Costs With and Without the Intervention

| Time | Without intervention | | With intervention | | | Cost-savings |
	Medical costs	Total	Medical costs	Program**	Total	(Italics)
Baseline	$100,000	$100,000	$100,000	$0	$100,000	
Inflation*	1.05%		1.025%			
6 months	$105,000	$105,000	$102,500	$7,500	$110,000	$5,000
12 months	$110,250	$110,250	$105,062	$7,500	$112,562	$2,312
18 months	$115,762	$115,762	$107,689	$7,500	$115,189	*($573)*
24 months	$121,550	$121,550	$110,381	$7,500	$117,881	*($3,669)*
30 months	$127,628	$127,628	$113,140	$7,500	$120,640	*($6,987)*
36 months	$134,009	$134,009	$115,969	$7,500	$123,469	*($10,540)*
42 months	$140,710	$140,710	$118,868	$7,500	$126,368	*($14,341)*
48 months	$147,745	$147,745	$121,840	$7,500	$129,340	*($18,405)*
Net savings					$ 47,203	

*Adjusted to reflect six months inflation; annual inflation is twice this percentage.
**Adjusted to reflect the six months cost of programming; annual cost is $15,000.

Break-Even Analysis

Break-even analysis (BEA) is a specialized version of forecasting and often provides evaluators with a more precise way of doing forecasting because, unlike plain forecasting, it makes an effort to take all possible costs and benefits into account. Although BEA is particularly applicable in evaluation situations that warrant a close inspection of specific benefits and costs, general forecasting is often a more viable option when evaluators have broadly defined benefits and costs to use in their evaluations.

Various measurement tools are available for determining the financial success or liability of a health promotion intervention, but some evaluators believe that none is more powerful than break-even analysis. BEA is a specialized application of forecasting techniques that enables you to estimate fairly accurately when the break-even point (when benefits and costs are of equal value) will be reached. It offers decision makers a clear way to determine if a specific intervention is on the right track. Sometimes referred to as **cost-volume-profit analysis** or **contribution analysis**, BEA can help decision makers answer key questions such as the following:

- Will a program or facility generate benefits which equal or exceed costs?
- How long will I have to wait to see a positive return on my investment?
- How many positive outcomes must people experience for the company to produce a profit?

As the demand for greater accountability and tighter budgets intensifies, program planners should know the operating status of their programs and services. There should be a clear understanding of which are profitable and which are not. As new programs are considered, well-informed decisions can be made only after determining the potential profitability of these offerings. Certainly not all programs and services are established to generate a direct profit; nonetheless, program directors and decision makers should understand where the break-even point is and what factors influence how quickly it occurs. A typical break-even graph is shown in figure 4.15.

Preliminary Steps for BEA

The first step in performing a BEA is to identify, measure, and calculate the monetary value of all cost items. A simple form such as the one shown in figure 4.16 provides a good structure for listing the monthly totals of the cost categories you will need to add up once you begin the BEA.

The second step is to add fixed and variable costs to calculate total costs (figure 4.17) using the following formula:

$$\text{Total costs} = \text{fixed costs} + \text{variable costs}$$

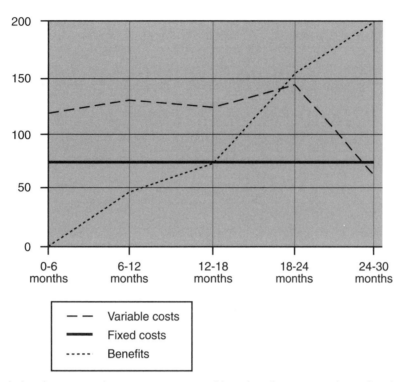

Figure 4.15 This sample break-even graph comparing costs and benefits of a program shows that the total of fixed and variable costs will equal the benefits after about 30 months.

	Jan.	**Feb.**	**March**	**April**	**May**	**June**	*Total*
Fixed							
Salaries							
Rent							
Insurance							
Property tax							
Depreciation							
Other:							
Variable							
Staff wages							
Utilities							
Phone/fax							
HRAs							
Equipment							
Other:							

Figure 4.16 A sample six-month expense record form.

	Jan.	Feb.	March	April	May	June	*Total*
Fixed							
Salaries	$150,000	$150,000	$150,000	$150,000	$150,000	$150,000	$900,000
Rent	2,700	2,700	2,700	2,700	2,700	2,700	16,200
Insurance	1,400	1,400	1,400	1,400	1,400	1,400	1,400
Property tax	1,500	1,500	1,500	1,500	1,500	1,500	900
Depreciation	1,000	1,000	1,000	1,000	1,000	1,000	6,000
Other:							
							$939,600
Variable							
Staff wages	$12,000	$14,500	$11,000	$13,800	$14,100	$12,300	$77,700
Utilities	3,400	3,500	3,300	3,100	2,900	2,750	18,950
Phone/fax	190	180	197	198	204	200	1,169
HRAs	2,000	0	0	0	0	0	2,000
Equipment	2,300	2,400	0	1,000	0	1,500	7,200
Other:							
							$107,019
						Combined total:	$1,046,619

Figure 4.17   A completed six-month expense record.

The Baseline and the Benefit Variable

The third step involves two procedures. The first is to determine a baseline so you will have a reference against which to project future costs and benefits. The second procedure is to determine a benefit variable (sometimes called a **tangible benefit**) to compare against fixed and variable costs identified earlier.

Establishing the Baseline

Since BEA involves some degree of forecasting, it is important to establish a valid baseline or reference point upon which to base your projections. Refer back to the discussion of establishing a baseline for simple forecasting (pages 98-100).

Calculating a Benefit Variable

Once you have an established baseline to serve as your reference point, you need to decide how to properly calculate a benefit variable.

The benefit variable should reflect one or more of the primary goals associated with each intervention. For example, if the main goals of your low back injury prevention program are

- to reduce the number of low back injuries and
- to reduce the average cost of low back injuries,

your corresponding benefit variables would be

- number of low back injuries and
- average cost of low back injury.

The best way to calculate a benefit variable for a BEA is to compute and compare future injuries and costs without the intervention (based on past trends) with future injuries and costs with an intervention, the latter being based on the initial impact of the intervention being evaluated.

To proceed with our low back injury example, let's assume that low back injury costs have risen 5% every three months for the past year. Your intervention has been underway for three months, and it has reduced low back injury-related medical care costs by 20% during that time. Projecting the future is, of course, an iffy enterprise. But, even while acknowledging that the unexpected may happen, one can make reasonable assumptions by looking carefully at factors that could influence the outcome, such as the following:

- The figures quoted above
- The fact that more employees will be brought into the program over time
- The expectation that employees in the program will report their low back injuries earlier than they did before they were in the program, resulting in their injuries being less severe, and thus less costly to treat than previous injuries

The evaluator feels safe in assuming that the 20% savings will be repeated every quarter for the next 21 months. She projects how the trend established during the three-month intervention will play out during that time period (see table 4.7).

Every forecasting scenario, no matter how meticulously prepared, is subject to many factors that will influence its accuracy. Note that the evaluator of table 4.7 has done more than take the data into account; she has included other factors, such as more employees being brought in and injuries being reported earlier. It is important that, like this evaluator, you brainstorm about factors beyond the data. For example, is the program already covering the departments where low back injuries are most

Table 4.7   A Comparison of Low Back Injury Claims and Costs With and Without an Intervention

| Interval | With intervention* | | Without intervention** | |
	Cost ($)	Claims (#)	Cost ($)	Claims (#)
Baseline	100,000	200	100,000	200
0-3 months	80,000	180	105,000	210
4-6 months	64,000	160	110,250	220
7-9 months	51,200	150	115,762	220
10-12 months	40,960	130	121,550	230
13-15 months	32,760	120	127,628	240
16-18 months	26,210	110	134,009	240
19-21 months	20,970	100	140,710	250

*(based on initial 20% impact)
**(based on past trend of 5% increase per year)

common, or are these departments yet to be included? Are you including publicity about positive results and expecting that this publicity will bring more participants into the program? Is the nature of the intervention such that its benefits will level off for participants after, say, one year of supervised exercise, and how will this affect the bottom line? In any case, because uncertainty characterizes most forecasting situations, short-term projections carry less risk for evaluators than making long-term (multiyear) projections.

Calculate Current and Projected Benefits

The fourth step is to calculate projected benefits (in dollars) based on any cost-reduction. For example, using the comparative low back injury (LBI) cost data in table 4.7, you can see that cost-savings per quarter with the intervention would be as shown in table 4.8.

If the annual cost of running the low back injury prevention program is $45,000, we can see from table 4.8 that, if the projected benefits are correct, the cost-reduction value would offset the program costs (break even) early in the second quarter. Even if there were little or no continuing impact from the program, it would have paid for itself before midyear. Now suppose that annual program costs were $100,000 and that the intervention impact could be sustained throughout the entire year. How long would it take for savings to offset the cost of the program in that case? At the sustained 20% impact rate, cost-savings would offset the program costs at approximately the eighth month, or about midway in the third quarter. If your initial impact is not as dramatic as those in our low back injury example, you should use actual cost-differences over two or more consecutive time frames to verify any assumption before making your break-even prediction.

Note the significant differences between the quarterly and cumulative cost-differences. It is important to decide the best way to use and illustrate these cost-differences in your BEA report. You have at least two viable options to consider:

- Treat cost-differences on an interval basis (e.g., quarterly, semiannually, annually), listing costs per year.
- Treat cost-differences on a cumulative basis, adding interval-to-interval differences. The advantages and disadvantages of each of these choices are discussed in chapter 6.

Calculate the Break-Even Point

The fifth step is to illustrate the break-even point. This can be done in several ways. One way is to draw a graph in which the intervention cost line intersects the cost-

Table 4.8 Program-Generated Savings

Time frame	LBI costs with intervention	LBI costs without intervention	Program-generated savings Quarterly	Cumulative
0-3 months	$80,000	$105,000	$25,000	$ 25,000
4-6 months	$64,000	$110,250	$46,250	$ 71,250
7-9 months	$51,200	$115,762	$64,562	$135,812
10-12 months	$40,960	$121,550	$80,590	$216,402

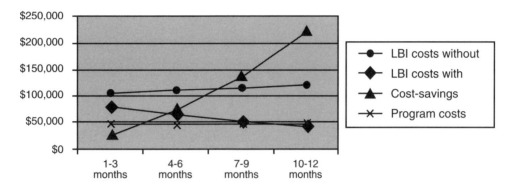

Figure 4.18 A BEA projection of low back injury costs without the program, with the program, and cumulative cost-savings at quarterly intervals. Note that the program costs $45,000 for the year, not per quarter.

savings (benefit) line at the break-even point as shown in figure 4.18. Bar charts and contrasting linear grids may also be used, but these alternatives are discussed in detail in chapter 6.

Penetration Impact Formula

The preceding steps serve as the mechanical basis for preparing and calculating a break-even analysis. However, the mechanics alone don't address other questions that decision makers need to take into account. For example, what level of participation is needed to achieve a break-even point? What degree of impact is sufficient to bring benefits on par with costs? How much do intervention costs need to be cut if participation or impact levels are less than expected? As long as the costs of the risk factors involved are known, a formula known as **penetration impact** can yield information of great value in answering these questions.

How many at-risk employees does your health management intervention have to reach and affect to pay for itself? That depends primarily on three factors:

1. The cost of the intervention
2. The individual (unit) cost of the targeted risk factor or health claim (RF cost)
3. The number of participants who successfully achieve the intervention goal

By factoring in each of these influences, the penetration impact formula can indicate what level of impact and effectiveness your intervention needs to achieve to reach the break-even point. For example, suppose you plan to spend $5,000 of your health management budget to reduce the number of at-risk employees with a specific risk factor. Suppose your risk factor cost appraisal (chapter 3) has indicated the risk factor is $200 per at-risk employee. Based on this scenario, a penetration impact can be conducted using the following equation, which would show that the intervention would need to affect at least 25 at-risk individuals for the cost-savings to equal/offset the intervention cost (see figure 4.19). This tool can be applied to virtually any situation as long as the intervention cost and unit cost (e.g., risk factor) are known.

$$\$5,000 \div \$200 = 25$$

Although a break-even analysis can be powerful tool for program planners to determine the financial potential of a new service, program, or facility, it should not take the place of market analysis, personnel decisions, planning, or other essential processes. Used correctly and in conjunction with other analysis techniques,

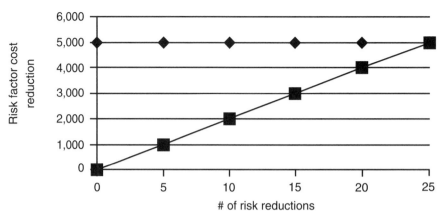

Figure 4.19 Graphing a penetration impact equation.

break-even analysis can yield valuable information for decision makers to use in making sound health management decisions.

Cost-Effectiveness Analysis

What if you want to compare three intervention programs with one another to determine which one produces the greatest benefit for the least expense? When properly designed and implemented, a cost-effectiveness analysis (CEA) can answer such a question. A CEA is a measure of the cost of an intervention relative to its impact, usually expressed in dollars per unit of effect.

A cost-effective intervention is one that achieves a health objective at less cost than alternative interventions. If you want to determine which of two smoking cessation interventions is the most cost-effective by using CEA, you could come up with figures that could be compared, as in table 4.9.

Rather than assigning monetary values to a single intervention outcome (as is done in some analyses), cost-effectiveness analysis compares only the costs of alternate interventions for achieving a specific outcome, measured in whatever units happen to be appropriate. This approach avoids the difficult issues of having to measure indirect benefits. It also allows for comparisons of marginal and average costs of given physical outcomes. In some cases, a CEA approach may point to the lowest cost alternative for a procedure that shows little or no net benefit in other analyses.

Considering the results shown in table 4.9, you could conclude that the cold turkey approach was less costly to offer and three times more economical (or one-third as costly to produce a positive outcome) than the gradual withdrawal approach.

There are limitations to using CEA approaches in program evaluation, however. One obvious shortcoming is that sometimes such an analysis does not lead to any clear-cut decision. This is the case when comparing two programs in which one is either less costly but also less effective or more costly but also more effective than the

Table 4.9 A Cost-Effectiveness Analysis Framework Used in Comparing Two Different Smoking Cessation Interventions

Intervention	Cost of program	Participants (# of)	Cost per participant	Quitters	Cost per quitter*
"Cold turkey" with self-help booklet	$2,000	100	$20	50	$ 40
Gradual withdrawal with on-site counseling	$3,000	100	$30	25	$120

*Cost of program divided by number of quitters

other. Similarly, when a particular intervention generates more value at less expense than its competitor, yet only a few employees are willing to participate in the more successful program, a CEA alone may not tell you which program is the best one to offer. This problem can occasionally be solved using efficiency criteria, such as choosing based on the amount of effect per unit of cost. Additional criticisms that are not as readily resolved include ambiguity regarding what program outcomes to emphasize and what costs to include. Other problems include selecting appropriate discount rates and other cost estimation methods when predictions are being made. (A discount rate is a quantitative index that is used to determine the future value of current costs and benefits. See *Determining Present Versus Future Value*, page 122 for further discussion of discount rates).

Eeeny, Meeny, Meiny, Mo

It is often the case that a single evaluation technique will not provide sufficient information for decision making. Suppose, for example, that a worksite offers two versions of a weight management program. One version consists only of an exercise program while the other version consists of an exercise program and a nutrition component. Both interventions have 50 participants and are offered for eight weeks. The employer's cost to offer the exercise-only program is $1,000 and produces a group weight loss of 416 pounds, or $2.40 per pound lost. In contrast, the employer's cost to offer the exercise/nutrition program is $3,000, but it produces a group weight loss of 1,200 pounds, or $2.50 per pound lost. Overall, the less costly program produced less weight loss than the higher cost program, which produced significantly more weight loss. Yet, the CEA ratios ($2.40 vs. $2.50) are virtually identical, indicating that neither of these interventions was clearly more cost-effective. Having completed their CEA, the evaluators will have to make use of further tools.

Performing a CEA

Performing a cost-effectiveness analysis in an organizational setting can be simplified with a clear-cut action plan. Table 4.10 illustrates a step-by-step approach for designing and implementing a CEA.

1. Plan your evaluation as you plan your interventions.
   - Determine your program's goal and objectives. Ask yourself what your interventions are supposed to do for employees or the organization. For example, the goal of the back program is to prevent low back injuries. Objectives listed in figure 4.20 represent several activities that must be

Table 4.10 Costing Items in CEA

Facilities

Cost item	Typically . . .	Occasionally . . .
Existing facilities	No	
Fitness center	No	If a substantial portion of the center is frequently used and other nonfitness activities have to be moved or rescheduled
Clinical settings	No	If off-site and contracted (rented, leased)
Meeting rooms exclusively	No	If rooms were built or designated for a program
Counseling center	No	If off-site and contracted (rented, leased)

Equipment and materials

Cost item	Typically . . .	Occasionally . . .
Fitness equipment	Yes	If leased or rented for a specified time
Screening equipment	Yes	If leased or rented for a specified time
Audiotapes, books, booklets, brochures, health risk appraisals	No	If purchased or used for the intervention
Hotlines and other phone-based services	Yes	
Photocopying	No	

Personnel

Cost item	Typically . . .	Occasionally . . .
Full-time staff	Yes	
Part-time staff	Yes	

Worktime

Cost item	Typically . . .	Occasionally . . .
Any scheduled worktime used for program participants	Yes	

accomplished to achieve the goal. For example, the first and second objectives include screening as many employees as possible to identify those at risk of incurring a low back injury. The third objective is to recruit and involve as many at-risk employees as possible in the year-long program. The fourth and final objective is to obtain feedback from participants as to whether or not they had incurred a low back injury. The final objective listed in a CEA framework should relate specifically to the main goal of the intervention.

- Set up thorough record keeping procedures. Consider major cost items such as personnel, facilities, equipment, and minor cost items such as duplicating and record keeping. You can use the Sample CEA Worksheet (page 115) for CEA as well as BEA. It is important to decide which items should be factored into the analysis. For example, since most on-site fitness facilities are physically housed inside or connected to other worksite buildings, organizations typically consider heating, cooling, and other utility costs as an incidental cost and thus do not charge these costs to the fitness center budget. Use table 4.10 as a guide when considering which cost items should be factored into a CEA.

- Determine the time frame during which you will compare your interventions.

2. Calculate total costs for each intervention. During the trial period, keep careful records following the procedures you instituted in step one. At the end of the trial period, add up all expenses to arrive at the total cost for each intervention during that period. To compare programs, enter that total in a worksheet like *A Sample CEA Worksheet* on page 115. You may copy and use the worksheet for this purpose.

3. Determine the cost per outcome for each program intervention. The cost per outcome is determined by dividing the cost of the program intervention by the number of quantitative units listed within each objective.

4. Compare the final cost per outcome values for each program intervention and determine which is most cost-effective. Two interventions designed to prevent low back injuries are compared in figure 4.20. You can see that not only did the seminar/lumbar belt intervention initially cost more in absolute terms than the daily prework stretching intervention, but also the prework stretching intervention was far more cost effective ($60 to prevent a low back injury versus $135 for the seminar/lumbar belt intervention). Similarly, table 4.9 compares the cost effectiveness of two smoking cessation projects. Clearly, the simpler intervention is the most cost-effective in both cases.

Goal: To prevent low back injuries

	Program A Monthly back seminar/ lumbar belt Annual cost: $5,000	Program B Daily prework stretch Annual cost: $3,000
Objective	Cost per outcome	Cost per outcome
Provide low back screens	$50 per screen*	$50 per screen*
Diagnose high risk workers	50 diagnosed at $100 per finding of high risk for low back injury	80 diagnosed at $37.50 per finding of high risk for low back injury
Retain as many participants as possible	$125 per completion (40)	$40 per completion (75)
Achieve injury-free status in participants	37 reported no low back injury during one year program: $135 per injury-free case	50 reported no low back injury during one year program: $60 per injury-free case

Figure 4.20 A cost-effectiveness analysis of two worksite back programs. The goal is to prevent low back injuries. (*The screening protocol used in both programs was identical.)

Although a CEA may show one intervention having a greater return-on-investment (ROI), than another, the decision to keep or eliminate a particular health management intervention should not be based solely on this comparison. After all, an intervention with a moderate ROI may produce certain benefits that are considered the following:

- Not easily quantified—for example, enhanced employee morale
- Not experienced throughout an organization—for example, fewer accidents that lead to greater productivity in some departments but not in others
- Delayed—for example, enhanced management-labor relations that reduce the prospect of a damaging labor strike

Looking Below the Surface gives a clear example of a situation that warranted retaining a program that appeared to have a low ROI when analyzed by CEA. The benefits in such situations may not show up on a CEA, but they can make an enormous positive difference in the atmosphere and even the bottom line of an organization. Thus, while it is important to know the data about cost-effectiveness, evaluators must bear in mind that such data are only part of the evidence they must look at when considering questions of program retention.

Looking Below the Surface

After experiencing 20% annual increases in mental health claims over the past five years, a large utility services company established an in-house employee assistance program (EAP) and a telephone-based counseling hotline. Health management personnel designed the EAP for immediate access by the company's 800 on-site employees and contracted a nationwide mental health provider to provide the hotline service to the 250 off-site workers. The total operating fees charged by both providers were substantially less than the mental health claims the company had been paying for. Both interventions were launched on January 1 with the dual goal of

- providing top quality and immediate mental health counseling to employees in need and
- reducing the demand on outside mental health providers.

Procedures were established to track mental health usage of the EAP and the hotline at quarterly intervals and mental health claims at six months and year-end. Midyear tracking data indicated that approximately 5% of all in-house employees were using the on-site EAP. In contrast, the hotline services were used by only 1% of all eligible off-site employees. Cost-wise, a single EAP counseling session was $15 compared to $50 for a single hotline session. This sharp contrast suggested the off-site hotline service was not as cost-effective as the EAP.

Upon reviewing this disparity, decision makers contemplated the possible elimination of the hotline service but decided to postpone this decision for several reasons. First, if the contract was terminated prematurely by the company, they would have to pay a huge penalty to the hotline provider. Second, they suspected that unknown barriers might be preventing off-site employees from using the hotline services very much.

Finally, they realized that many of the off-site workers were some of the most loyal and experienced employees within the entire organization. In hopes of getting a clearer picture of the situation, the company administered a questionnaire to all off-site employees asking them to identify what factors were preventing them from using the hotline. Nearly 75% of the off-site employees responded, and their answers provided some unexpected and startling results—over 50% of the off-site employees were not even aware that the hotline service

(continued)

existed! Apparently there had been a major miscommunication between the employer and hotline provider that resulted in this marketing fiasco. Both parties quickly expanded their marketing efforts to increase employee awareness of the hotline. Follow-up tracking efforts revealed that a growing number of off-site employees were using the hotline services throughout the third and fourth quarters. CEA evaluations showed that the cost of a single hotline counseling session had dropped to a more competitive rate of $20 per encounter, only slightly more than the cost of an EAP session. Because of this enhanced performance, the company decided to maintain the hotline service, and they now anticipate even greater results in the future.

The *Sample CEA Worksheet* on this page can be customized to fit your evaluation plans. This sample format is designed to compare two interventions. If you want to compare three or more interventions, simply add more *Cost per outcome* columns to reflect the number of interventions being evaluated.

Using CEA to Forecast Value

In addition to measuring the current value of multiple interventions, the CEA procedure can be modified to forecast the future value of current programs. For example, let's assume decision makers want to know the cost-effectiveness of treating minor acute illnesses or accidents by an occupational health nurse at the worksite versus seeking treatment off-site at a doctor's office or hospital emergency department. The first step is to construct a CEA worksheet that is customized to track the scope and specificity of cost items that are readily available/accessible to evaluation personnel. For example, if evaluators do not have access to the costs of prescription drugs, equipment, utilities, and so forth, their CEA tool would be constructed as

A Sample CEA Worksheet

Goal:_____

Objective	Program A $ _____ (cost) Cost per outcome	Program B $ _____ (cost) Cost per outcome
o_____	$_____	$_____
o_____	$_____	$_____
o_____	$_____	$_____
o_____ *	$_____ *	$_____ *

*Reflects goal

shown in figure 4.21. A fact that evaluators must keep in mind in this case is that over 50% of all emergency department visits are actually nonemergencies that do not require the services of an off-site health care provider.

Here is a set of procedures for using CEA to forecast the value of retaining an occupational health nurse. Figure 4.21 shows the calculations involved in the on-site and off-site options:

I. First, ask preliminary questions to determine whether the question is worth pursuing. In this case, the steps would be as follows:

1. Using CDA, count the total number of nonemergency situations on which the company spent money the previous year.

2. Estimate what percentage of a full-time position would need to be devoted to treating that many minor ailments.

3. Decide whether there are essential tasks that could be done by the nurse in the time that would be left over (employee education, employee health evaluations, paperwork, meetings).

4. In the light of your answers, decide whether to proceed with the CEA. In this case, the evaluator concluded that the nurse would average treating one minor ailment per hour (eight per day) and that approximately 45 minutes of every on-site hour would be devoted to nonacute duties such as employee health screening, environment testing, administrative paper work, data entry, and meetings.

II. Next, calculate the costs of on-site treatment.

1. List annual salary and benefits paid to health care provider (occupational health nurse): $44,800.

2. Determine and list the nurse's annual workload: 2,000 hours.

Occupational nurse:	On-site	vs.	Off-site	
Annual salary	$35,000		Visit to doctor's office or emergency department	$150
(Fringe benefits)	+ 9,800		(20% employee co-payment)	−30
Total	$44,800			$120
Annual workload	2,000 hrs			
Minutes per case:	× .25 hr (15 min)			
% of workload	.000125			
	×44,800			
Labor cost per case	$5.60			

Unit cost difference: $114 ($120 − $5.60)

	Daily	Weekly	Monthly	Annually
Unit difference	$114	$912	$4,560	$18,240
× number of cases	× 8	× 5	× 4	× 12
Total	$912	$4,560	$18,240	$218,880

Figure 4.21   A sample cost-effectiveness analysis framework.

3. Determine and list the average number of minutes needed to treat a minor ailment: 15 (.25 hr).

4. Calculate the percentage of the health care provider's annual workload devoted exclusively to treating a single minor ailment: .000125. This was determined by dividing .25 by 2000.

5. Multiply the percentage of workload devoted to each case (.000125) by annual compensation ($44,800) to determine the company's labor cost to treat one minor ailment ($5.60).

III. Calculate the costs of off-site treatment.

1. Determine and list the average outpatient claim cost incurred in a primary physician's office or emergency department: $150.00.

2. Determine the average out-of-pocket deductible or co-payment paid by the employee (**cost-share**): 20% (based on a health plan provision with no deductible and a 20% co-payment).

3. Multiply the employee's cost-share (.20) by the total charge ($150) to determine the employee's direct cost ($30) and subtract from the total charge to determine the employer's health care expense: $120.

4. Compare labor costs for on-site health care ($5.60) versus off-site health care ($120) to determine cost-difference (about $114, rounded off). This does not include indirect costs such as prescription medication, equipment costs, property taxes, and so on.

IV. Project future cost-avoidance benefits.

1. List cost-difference ($114) and multiply by the number of on-site ailments (8) to compute daily cost-avoidance ($912).

2. Multiply the daily cost-avoidance as follows to determine weekly, monthly, and annual cost-avoidance benefits:

	Daily	**Weekly**	**Monthly**	**Annually**
Unit Difference	$114	$ 912	$ 4,560	$ 18,240
× # of units	× 8 cases	× 5 days	× 4 wks	× 12 mo
	$ 912	$4,560	$18,240	$218,880

Based on the results of the process previously summarized (shown in detail in figure 4.21), the more cost-effective solution is for the organization to provide on-site health care services to treat acute (minor) ailments than to relinquish this care to off-site health care providers.

Because CEA is a good tool for comparing two or more interventions in terms of bang for the buck and because it can be used to look at either past performance or projections of future performance, it is a good technique to help objectively determine if a particular intervention should be continued, expanded, dropped, or revised.

REVIEW QUESTIONS: COST-EFFECTIVENESS ANALYSIS

1. What situations warrant a cost-effectiveness analysis?

2. What is the step-by-step process used to prepare and conduct a CEA?

3. How can a CEA be used to forecast value?

Benefit-Cost Analysis

While CEA is most useful for choosing the most efficient program from among various alternatives, benefit-cost analysis (BCA) is most useful for evaluating a single program. The essential difference between CEA and BCA is that CEA is primarily focused on the cost to achieve a specific effect while BCA primarily focuses on any and all benefits that can be generated for a program cost. To put it another way, cost-effectiveness is expressed as dollars per unit of effect (e.g., $10 for every new employee screened for a low back injury prevention program) while benefit-cost can be expressed as a ratio of total benefits achieved for every dollar spent on a program (e.g., $20 saved in emergency department visits not made and work time not lost for every dollar spent on a medical self-care program). The greater the number of benefits and costs that can be accurately measured in monetary terms, the more useful BCA will be. Although BCA is generally used to judge the value of a single intervention, its framework can also provide economic comparisons of two or more interventions.

BCA can be applied to a program during its planning stage (**ex ante**) or after it has been in operation (**ex post facto**). The major difference between the two approaches is that the former requires many more assumptions and cost estimates than does the latter. Since there are empirical data on actual costs and benefits in an ex post facto BCA, its results are usually far more accurate and reliable than those of an ex ante BCA. For an ex post facto analysis, the record of actual expenditures is used while for an ex ante analysis the proposed budget must be used.

Performing a Benefit-Cost Analysis

Because benefit-cost analysis provides meaningful data only to the extent that current or future benefits and costs can be accurately measured or projected, the first step in executing a BCA is to identify and measure benefits and costs as precisely as possible.

Identifying and Measuring Costs

The cost side of a benefit-cost analysis involves calculating the costs of all resources such as personnel, equipment, and facilities used in planning and implementing an intervention. Typical direct and indirect costs are shown in *Examples of Direct and Indirect Costs to Employers.*

Examples of Direct and Indirect Costs to Employers

Direct	Indirect (opportunity)
Medical care	Absenteeism (injured or sick employees)
Medical supplies	Additional tasks for coworkers
Medications, pharmacy services	Training of replaced workers
Rehabilitation	Supervision of replaced workers
Employee assistance	Lower productivity from replaced workers
Workers' compensation	Reduced performance of returning workers
Case management	Data processing/administration
Legal fees	Drug testing
Temporary worker payments	Regulatory compliance
Compliance with OSHA	Development of health and safety policies
ADA accommodations	Overtime pay
Involvement of other departments	Unexpected costs

The most difficult task in both ex ante and ex post facto BCA evaluations is to identify and calculate the impact of opportunity costs on employee and organizational health. The following are typical of situations in which opportunity costs occur:

- **Improper planning.** Suppose an organization simultaneously establishes an on-site recreation center and an in-house EAP, both of which generate twice as much employee demand as expected. Moreover, neither program is properly staffed, eventually leading to a significant drop-off in employee participation. As more employees' needs and interests go unmet, none of the goals originally established for either intervention is achieved; thus, there is a *lost opportunity* to make a positive impact.

- **Unexpected catastrophic events.** For example, a flu epidemic occurs during a company's peak production time and results in significant absenteeism throughout the workforce. The organization experiences not only a noticeable drop in production, but unexpected medical care costs and higher payroll costs to hire replacement workers as well.

- **Redistribution of resources.** Suppose an organization's on-site fitness center equipment begins to break down due to age, delayed maintenance, and heavy utilization. The fitness center budget does not include sufficient funds for repairing the broken equipment. Therefore, decision makers elect to tap the company's contingency fund to cover this huge expense, leaving limited resources for similar expenses in the future.

- **Inaccurate projections.** Suppose a work-life survey shows strong employee interest in wellness days off and healthier cafeteria food. In response, the organization renegotiates its food service contract for the vendor to provide heart-healthy entrees. Simultaneously, the organization establishes a wellness days off policy for employees meeting designated participation levels. Policy makers project that approximately 20% of all employees will qualify for the days off. Surprisingly, nearly 40% of all employees qualify for the incentive within two months, and as expected, many take their days off in the same month. Organizational productivity drops to a historic low, especially in departments with a high number of participants.

Identifying and Measuring Benefits

The benefit side of the equation involves calculating the monetary value of any positive outcomes that can be quantified. As with costs, it is necessary to take both direct and indirect benefits into account.

Indirect benefits are also often referred to as **opportunity benefits** because they represent a financial resource that unexpectedly becomes available to invest in other interventions. The author prefers the term **cost avoidance** benefits because an indirect benefit is the amount of future dollars not spent, rather than dollars actually saved and deposited. Moreover, costs that are not incurred can't be measured directly because they are not tangible.

Benefits, whether direct or indirect, include lower medical costs, fewer accidents, lower absenteeism, and higher productivity. The effects of direct benefits are usually measurable using standard accounting reports and conventional financial analysis. Before any direct benefit can be calculated, evaluators must identify an outcome (dependent) variable that can be treated as a direct benefit. In doing so, recall that a variable must be both measurable and related to the intervention. The effects of indirect benefits on profitability can be very large, though difficult to prove using conventional cost-accounting.

Comparing Costs and Benefits

After all costs and the value of all benefits have been identified and measured, the two categories are compared. To do this comparison, we use either the net benefit method or the benefit-cost ratio method.

The Net Benefit Method

In this method, the evaluator determines the **net benefit** of a particular intervention and compares that with its cost. If the difference is positive, the analysis indicates that the intervention is financially worth the effort.

The net benefit of any intervention may be calculated in the following manner:

$$\text{Net Benefit} = [\text{L\$} + \text{GP} + \text{PI}] - \text{C}$$

where

- L\$ (sometimes called the **direct benefit**) stands for the reduction in medical care expenses due to reduced disease or disability. For example, if the incidence of low back injury declines, then some of the spending on physicians and other medical care services will no longer be necessary and thus saved for the employee, employer, society, or other payers.
- GP stands for the increase in general productivity, leading to greater output and income. For example, if we reduce the incidence of low back injury, we also increase the performance capabilities of the persons involved so they may continue to produce at desirable levels.
- PI stands for the gain in working income due to reduced illness and injury and their effects on absenteeism (lost income). GP and PI are the indirect benefits.
- C stands for the cost of the intervention.

For example, suppose an organization is experiencing a significant increase in low back injury costs and responds by establishing a back injury prevention program. After six months of the program, evaluators conduct a benefit-cost analysis. To use the formula above, they need to find out the value of the reduction in medical care expenses related to low back, the increase in general productivity, and the drop in the cost of absenteeism. Here is what they find:

- Medical care expenses for back injures have dropped from $125,000 to $35,000, so L\$ = $90,000.
- Production output (as measured by the financial value of goods produced by employees) has increased by $35,000, so GP = $35,000.
- Employees' absenteeism due to illness and injury declined 2%, resulting in a drop of $4,000 in absentee expenses, so PI = $4,000.
- The cumulative program intervention cost for operating the program is $35,000, so C = $35,000.

If we apply the preceding data to the net benefit equation, it would be as follows:

$$\text{Net benefit} = [\$90{,}000 + \$35{,}000 + \$4{,}000] - \$35{,}000 = \$94{,}000$$

When one considers that the program has generated savings equal to almost three times its cost, the intervention clearly seems worth it.

The Benefit-Cost Ratio Method

The other most commonly used method is the benefit-cost ratio, calculated by dividing all program-related benefits by all program costs. That is,

$$B\,/\,C\ ratio = \frac{Benefit}{Cost}$$

For example, consider a hypertension control program that generated cost-avoidance savings of $50,000 via reduced hypertension-related absenteeism and hypertension-related health care costs, compared to an annual intervention cost of $20,000:

$$\frac{Benefit}{Cost} = \frac{\$50,000}{\$20,000} = \frac{\$2.50}{\$1.00}$$

Note that the final step is to divide both the upper and lower figures by the lower number. This calculation will always result in $1.00 as the unit of cost. Thus, in our example, a preliminary benefit-to-cost ratio of $50,000 to $20,000 would apply, and dividing both figures by $20,000 reveals that for every $1 of costs, $2.50 worth of benefits were achieved.

Of course, the preceding ratio can be compared to that of another program if evaluators want to determine which of the two programs is most cost-effective. For example, suppose the preceding program's benefit-cost ratio is compared with that of a low back program that yields the following ratio:

$$\frac{Benefit}{Cost} = \frac{\$20,000}{\$3,000} = \frac{\$6.66}{\$1.00}$$

Although both programs are successful, the back program produced a better benefit-to-cost ratio, and from an economic viewpoint, it is as important to the organization's health as the more expensive hypertension control program.

BCA Applied to Multiple Interventions

Another way to determine the net benefit of a single intervention or multiple interventions is illustrated in figure 4.22. It is a comparison of three types of medication used to treat migraine headaches. Using several **performance indicators** to reflect possible cost-savings, this example shows different BCA ratios based on medication costs versus reduced disability costs. The following is the procedure used to produce this table with the steps keyed to the numbers on the table:

1. List the number of persons participating in the intervention.
2. List the individual prescription cost, if known, or divide total prescription (R_x) cost by number of participants.
3. Multiply the number of participants by the annual cost per participant.
4. Calculate average number of days of work lost per person (disability days) per group.
   a. Divide the total number of disability days per group by the number of participants for a designated period of time (e.g., six months) before the intervention.
   b. Divide the total number of disability days per group by the number of participants during the intervention for the same time frame used for the *before* period.
   c. Subtract the number of disability days during the intervention from the number of disability days prior to the intervention.
5. Calculate the costs of the disability days and cost differences.
   a. Figure the total costs based on costs associated with job replacements and any measurable loss in actual productivity and divide that figure by the

total number of disability days to arrive at the average cost per disability day.

    b. Multiply average cost per disability day by the difference calculated in step 4c to arrive at the average cost per participant.

    c. Multiply cost difference per participant by number of participants to arrive at the total savings.

6. Divide any cost-savings (benefit) by the medication cost for each group to yield the benefit-cost ratio.

Whatever BCA approach is used, it is important to realize that the validity and reliability of any formula depends largely on the accuracy of the data used to quantify benefits and costs. The benefit-cost approach is typically used when one or two general categories of benefits and costs can be monetarily quantified. The net benefit BCA approach is typically used when only one or two types of benefit and cost data are available. In contrast, the third approach is commonly used when several types of benefit and cost data are available.

Determining Present Versus Future Value

Even when monetary values have been assigned to benefits and to direct and indirect costs, these values are not usually directly comparable because they occur over a period of time during which the **value of dollars** will most likely change.

	Medication		
	Brand A	Brand B	Brand C
1. Number of participants	50	50	50
2. Annual cost per participant	× $150	× $165	× $189
3. Total cost of medication	$7,500	$8,250	$9,450
Performance indicators			
4. Disability days (number per participant)			
a. Before	6.5	6.5	6.5
b. During	3.9	4.1	5.0
c. Difference	(−2.6)	(−2.4)	(−1.5)
5. Disability costs			
a. Average cost per disability	$200	$200	$200
b. Difference	× 2.6	× 2.4	× 1.5
c. Cost difference per participant	$520	$480	$300
d. Number of participants	× 50	× 50	× 50
e. Cost-difference (*savings*)	$26,000	$24,000	$15,000
Benefit-cost comparison			
6. Cost-difference (benefit)/ Cost of R$_x$ medicine	$26,000/ $7,500	$24,000/ $8,250	$15,000/ $9,450
7. Benefit-cost ratio	$3.47:1	$2.91:1	$1.59:1

Figure 4.22 A sample BCA framework.

Because dollars available today may be worth more or less than dollars available tomorrow, the present value of future dollars needs to be calculated to make reasonable dollar comparisons across different time periods. While this adjustment can be made in various ways, one of the most frequently used approaches involves choosing a discount rate that will be used in the formula for reducing future costs and benefits so they are comparable to the present value of money. Unfortunately, there are no standardized guidelines to follow in choosing a discount rate to be used in present value calculations. Many economists prefer to tie discount rates to the inflation rates associated with major cost items that are calculated. For example, if wages are rising annually at 4%, a discount rate of 4% would apply to personnel costs. Because present value calculations—as well as benefit-cost ratios and net gain or loss figures—are very sensitive to the discount rate chosen, an evaluator should conduct several analyses using different discount rates to determine how an intervention would fare under each rate. For example, a range of low-end to high-end discount rates may be used to represent possible best-case and worst-case scenarios. Suppose an organization is in the midst of trying to determine what its current health care budget can purchase in the next three to five years. The organization has been told by various benefits consultants that health care inflation is expected to rise 9% to 12% per year during this time frame. In an attempt to determine the full spectrum of potentially good or bad outcomes, the organization elects to use various discount rates ranging from the low-end 9% to, say, 15% on the premise that actual health care inflation rates may exceed the consultants' estimates.

Once you have chosen the discount rate you can use the following **present value adjustment** (PVA) formula for calculating the present value of future costs:

$$PV_c = \frac{C_y}{(1+r)^y}$$

PV_c refers to the costs for the entire program figured in current dollar values; C_y refers to the program costs for each year in which they occur; r refers to the discount rate; y refers to the year. For example, if an organization were to invest $40,000 per year for three consecutive years in a worksite health promotion intervention in which the discount rate was 10%, the present value of the costs of the program would be calculated as follows:

$$PV_c = C_1 + C_2 + C_3$$

Begin by calculating the values of C_1, C_2, and C_3 as follows:

$$C_1 = \frac{\$40,000}{(1+r)} = \frac{40,000}{(1+.10)} = \frac{40,000}{1.10} = \$36,363.64$$

$$C_2 = \frac{\$40,000}{(1+r)^2} = \frac{40,000}{(1+.10)^2} = \frac{40,000}{1.21} = \$33,057.85$$

$$C_3 = \frac{\$40,000}{(1+r)^3} = \frac{40,000}{(1+.10)^3} = \frac{40,000}{(1.331)} = \$30,052.59$$

Add the values of C_1, C_2, and C_3 to arrive at the total present value of costs of the program over a three-year period:

$$PV_c = \$36,363.64 + 33,057.85 + 30,052.59 = \$99,474.08$$

The three-year cost of this intervention expressed in the value of today's dollars is $99,474.

Computing an Aggregate Adjusted Inflation (Discount) Rate

Establishing a discount rate that accurately reflects costs requires evaluators to understand that all cost items are not necessarily affected at the same rate of inflation. Likewise, various benefits may be influenced at different rates of inflation.

For instance, suppose an organization establishes an on-site walking facility for its employees to use before work, during breaks, or after work. The major cost items revealed in the annual budget include

- a part-time facility attendant,
- several pieces of stretching equipment,
- facility maintenance, and
- utilities.

In order to determine a single overall discount rate for the combined cost items, it is necessary to identify appropriate inflation rates for each of the cost items. For example, to determine an inflation rate assigned to the attendant, you have to first acknowledge that part-time personnel do, in fact, receive yearly wage or salary increases, and, assuming they do, you must treat the percentage increase as the rate of inflation. Equipment inflation data could be based on the expected life span of the equipment, depreciation, and the manufacturer's warranty and replacement guidelines. Maintenance inflation can be determined by the company's yearly cost increases to pay for maintenance personnel and supplies. Utilities inflation can be determined by consulting the local utility provider.

Next you need to determine the percentage of total costs for each of the four cost categories. Using this data for each cost item along with the inflation rates for each, the following framework can be used to compute an aggregate inflation (discount) rate:

Cost item	% of total costs	$\times$	Inflation rate	=	Cost item inflation

Fill in the data you have gathered on each item into the formula:

• Attendant	.50 (50%)		4%	2.00%
• Equipment	.25 (25%)		5%	1.25%
• Maintenance	.20 (20%)		6%	1.20%
• Utilities	.05 (5%)		5%	0.25%

Finally, add up the *Cost item inflation* column to yield the project's aggregate inflation rate: 4.70%.

Based on the preceding data, the aggregate adjusted inflation (discount) rate is 4.7%.

In contrast, determining an aggregate discount rate for benefits is more challenging because benefits are more difficult to separate into categories than are cost items. Thus, evaluators will typically assign equal credit to each of the benefits in a PVA. For instance, suppose the walking facility generated three measurable benefits:

- A reduced number of visits to the on-site health nurse
- Reduced medical costs for hypertension
- Reduced workers' compensation payments for muscular strains

(continued)

Specific inflation rates that would apply in this situation could be obtained in several ways. For instance, the inflation rate for the occupational health nurse could be obtained by reviewing yearly wage and salary increases for such personnel; the inflation rate for reduced medical costs could be tied to the current rate of medical inflation; and the inflation rate for workers' compensation payments could be obtained by determining the annual percentage increase in these payments for the past two to three years. The same formula used for costs is used for benefits after substituting *benefit* for *cost* throughout:

Benefit	% of total benefits	×	Inflation rate	=	Benefit inflation

Again, plug the data you have obtained on each item into the formula:

• Reduced visits	.33 (1/3)		4%		1.32%
• Reduced medical costs	.33 (1/3)		8%		2.64%
• Reduced workers' compensation payments	.33 (1/3)		6%		1.80%

And again, add up the *Benefit inflation* column to arrive at the aggregate inflation rate for all the benefits considered: 5.76%.

In addition to being useful for determining direct and indirect benefits, a present value adjustment can be used to calculate the present and future value of net benefit-cost ratios (see figure 4.23). The present value of benefits (PV_b) is calculated the same way as the present value of costs except that monetized program benefits (B_y) are substituted for program costs (C_y) in the formula. Just as in the case of costs, the computation of the present discounted value of an intervention (the value today of payments in the future) requires the use of a discount rate to reflect that future dollars have less value than today's dollars. For example, suppose your self-care program was evaluated and showed a benefit-cost ratio of $1,000 to $750—in other words, a return of $1.33 for every $1 spent. Nonetheless, you wonder if this 33% return on investment (ROI) will have any staying power in the future. Chances are, it won't. The main reason is that the actual monetary value of dollars tied to benefits differs over time from that of dollars tied to costs. Thus, it is important to discount each of these values according to how the economy affects them. To do so, these values are subjected to different discount rates when the net benefit-cost ratios of the program are calculated (figure 4.23).

In figure 4.23, 10% has been chosen as the discount rate for the value of benefits. This is based on the fact that a discount rate of 5% to 10% has historically been used to depreciate the future value of an organization's health care cost-savings because corporate health care costs have risen annually in this range over the past decade. In this example, a discount rate of 10% was used to represent the high-end of the typical range because the evaluator believed that health care inflation in the future would actually be higher than the norm.

On the cost side, dollars spent to fund a health promotion intervention are weighed less heavily than future benefits for at least two reasons:

• First, due to inflation, a dollar can usually purchase more risk-reduction resources this year than it can next year.

1. Benefits

$$PV_b = \sum \frac{B_y}{(1+r)^y} = \frac{B_1}{(1+r)^1} + \frac{B_2}{(1+r)^2} + \frac{B_3}{(1+r)^3}$$

$$\frac{B_1}{(1+r)^1} = \frac{\$9{,}760}{(1+.10)^1} = \frac{\$9{,}760}{1.10^1} = \frac{\$9{,}760}{1.10} = \$8{,}872.73 \text{ (year 1)}$$

$$\frac{B_2}{(1+r)^2} = \frac{\$9{,}760}{(1+.10)^2} = \frac{\$9{,}760}{1.10^2} = \frac{\$9{,}760}{1.21} = \$8{,}066.12 \text{ (year 2)}$$

$$\frac{B_3}{(1+r)^3} = \frac{\$9{,}760}{(1+.10)^3} = \frac{\$9{,}760}{1.10^3} = \frac{\$9{,}760}{1.331} = \$7{,}332.83 \text{ (year 3)}$$

$$\sum \frac{B_y}{(1+r)^y} = \$8{,}872.73 + \$8{,}066.11 + \$7{,}332.83 = \$24{,}271.67$$

$PV_b = \$24{,}271.67$

2. Costs

Determine the approximate amount of personnel time devoted exclusively to screen, educate, and monitor (SEM) high-risk employees. The calculation for the cost of SEM time is the amount of the annual budget ($168,875.00) multiplied by the SEM time (4.5% of total workload).

Annual budget	$168,875.00
× SEM time	0.045
SEM cost to employer	**$7,599.38**

$$PV_c = \sum \frac{C_y}{(1+r)^y} = \frac{C_1}{(1+r)^1} + \frac{C_2}{(1+r)^2} + \frac{C_3}{(1+r)^3}$$

$$\frac{C_1}{(1+r)^1} = \frac{\$7{,}599.37}{(1+.075)^1} = \frac{\$7{,}599.37}{1.075^1} = \frac{\$7{,}599.37}{1.075} = \$7{,}069.18 \text{ (year 1)}$$

$$\frac{C_2}{(1+r)^2} = \frac{\$7{,}599.37}{(1+.075)^2} = \frac{\$7{,}599.37}{1.075^2} = \frac{\$7{,}599.37}{1.15} = \$6{,}608.15 \text{ (year 2)}$$

$$\frac{C_3}{(1+r)^3} = \frac{\$7{,}599.37}{(1+.075)^3} = \frac{\$7{,}599.37}{1.075^3} = \frac{\$7{,}599.37}{1.24} = \$6{,}128.52 \text{ (year 3)}$$

$$\sum \frac{C_y}{(1+r)^y} = \$7{,}069.18 + \$6{,}608.15 + \$6{,}128.52 = \$19{,}805.85$$

$PV_c = \$19{,}805.85$

3. Calculate net benefit-cost ratios

	Year 1	Year 2	Year 3
Benefit	$8,872.73	$8,066.11	$7,332.83
Cost	$7,069.18	$6,608.15	$6,128.52
Return on investment (ROI ratio)	$1.26 / $1.00	$1.22 / $1.00	$1.20 / $1.00

Figure 4.23 A sample present value adjustment framework.

- Second, economists depreciate the value of cost dollars at a lower discount rate than benefit dollars because intervention (cost) dollars could actually be deposited in a bank today and accrue a higher dividend than benefit dollars which cannot be deposited until they are achieved. Thus, cost dollars are invested for a longer time frame and consequently yield a larger return.

In addition, discount rates assigned to typical cost items are usually 25% to 50% lower than discount rates assigned to benefits. Hence, the costs in figure 4.23 have had a discount rate of 7.5% applied to them.

Notice that the ROI ratio in figure 4.23 gradually drops over time (from $1.26 to $1.20 in three years) because benefit dollars (discounted at 10%) depreciate faster than cost dollars (discounted at 7.5%). Thus, the current ROI will eventually disappear if the self-care program merely sustains the initial impact and fails to improve (see figure 4.24). The prospect of such shrinking ROIs causes many decision makers to ask the question, *Could we have invested the cost dollars in a different project and earned a higher ROI?* An organization could answer this question by using a cost-effectiveness analysis (CEA) to compare two different self-care programs against each other or to compare the self-care program against an unrelated program. In either case, the CEA could reveal which of the two interventions generated the most benefit for the least cost.

To summarize, BCA is an excellent tool for comparing the value of a program's costs and benefits, provided that all cost and benefit items can be reasonably measured and assigned monetary values. It is also important to incorporate present-value adjustment (PVA) formulas when possible, keeping in mind that the value of today's benefits and costs are affected differently by the marketplace. The information provided by a well-done BCA can be invaluable to decision makers as they plan for the future.

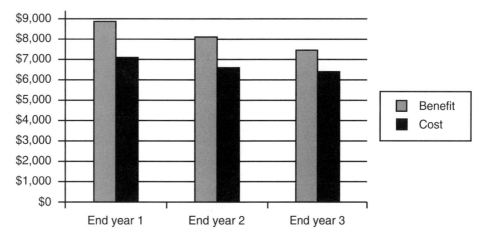

Figure 4.24   Declining benefit-cost ratios. Observe that the benefits and costs lines are beginning to converge.

REVIEW QUESTIONS: BENEFIT-COST ANALYSIS

1. What situations warrant a benefit-cost analysis?
2. How does a BCA differ from a cost-effectiveness analysis?
3. What is the step-by-step process used to prepare and conduct a BCA?
4. What purpose(s) does a present value adjustment (PVA) serve?

CHAPTER REVIEW

Summary

Various econometric analysis instruments are suitable for worksite health promotion evaluations. Forecasting, break-even analysis, cost-effectiveness analysis, and benefit-cost analysis offer evaluators varying degrees of versatility for determining the financial value of a stand-alone intervention, head-to-head intervention comparisons, and multiple intervention comparisons. Decision makers should carefully consider various factors before selecting any econometric tool. When properly incorporated into a sound evaluation framework by qualified evaluators, econometric analyses can produce valuable information for planning personnel to use in making well-informed decisions on which programs to eliminate, revise, and add.

Questions

1. What is the major difference between non-econometric and econometric tools for data analysis?

2. When is an appropriate time to conduct a forecast? A break-even analysis? A cost-effectiveness analysis? A benefit-cost analysis?

3. What are several examples of fixed costs? Variable costs?

4. What is a major difference between benefit-cost analysis and cost-effectiveness analysis?

5. What are the major components of a forecast?

6. What are the major steps used in preparing a forecast?

7. What is one situation in which you would use a forecast rather than a break-even analysis?

What Would You Do?

1. You have recently been asked to develop a tool to evaluate the potential cost-difference between an on-site medical self-care program provided by in-house staff versus a program provided by an outside firm. After identifying and quantifying all cost items for each option, you propose to your supervisor that a cost-effectiveness analysis (CEA) be used. She prefers that you do a projected benefit-cost analysis on each of the two options. Considering that this is a proposal, you steadfastly feel the CEA is a superior approach. To persuade her, what would you say?

2. Suppose a new ergonomics program has been operational for the past six months and has just been subjected to its first evaluation. The results show substantial decreases in selected musculoskeletal claims and costs, yet programming costs still exceed these cost-savings. Thus, your boss has asked you to conduct a break-even analysis (BEA) to determine when the program's benefits (reduced musculoskeletal claim costs) will offset the program's operational costs. Moreover, he wants a detailed BEA to incorporate specific types of musculoskeletal claim costs by ICD code. You explain that the organization's musculoskeletal claims data are generically formatted only by major diagnostic category (MDC). Consequently, you suggest that a forecast is more suitable due to the lack of ICD-coded cost data. He rejects this idea and contends that a BEA is the only way to go. To help him see the value of using a simple forecast in this situation, what would you say?

3. Your boss asks you to establish a plan to evaluate the in-house intranet health promotion delivery system. You are concerned that an evaluation of the system (which is only three months old) may be premature and that no goals were initially established for the program. Nonetheless, you propose a **graduated evaluation** in which one or two health-related outcome measurements would be conducted immediately to serve as a baseline, followed by several financial outcome measurements at quarterly intervals over the next nine months. Your boss estimates the program's first-year operating costs will be around $150,000 due primarily to the up-front intranet installation cost. After the first year, operating costs will be minimal. You have also been told that the company is experiencing a tight cash-flow situation, resulting in stricter cost-justification measures being invoked throughout the company. Your boss fears that the intranet program must pay for itself or face elimination. Considering the size of your organization (450 employees) and considering that approximately 20% of the workforce use the system at least once a week, you are concerned that the program cannot save $150,000 in the next nine months. Taking all of these factors into account, you rethink the merits of your initial proposal. You decide to suggest to your boss that he try to buy more time from management because you do not believe that the short-term time frame of nine months will generate adequate cost-savings. He is at a loss as to how to approach management with your request. Knowing the fate of the program may rest on your suggestion, what would you recommend?

PART III

Planning, Conducting, and Presenting Evaluations

5
Planning and Conducting Evaluations

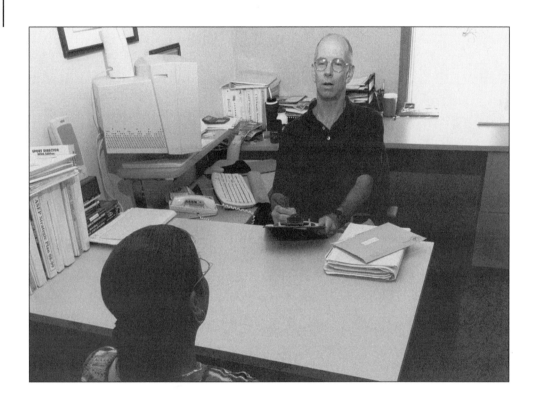

After reading this chapter and answering the questions at the end, you should be able to do the following:

- Identify various stakeholders and several ways to solicit their interest in an evaluation.
- Develop an evaluation goal that incorporates the five recommended criteria.
- Distinguish health-related goals and financial goals.
- List several dependent variables related to employees' health.
- Describe how to establish the scope and specificity of an evaluation.
- Determine when it is feasible to do a quantitative versus qualitative evaluation.
- Properly format specific types of data to enhance the quality of an analysis.

Now that we have looked at the types, basic procedures, and econometric and non-econometric instruments of worksite health promotion evaluation, it is time to learn how to incorporate all these elements into structures that will guide you through each step of evaluation. This chapter shows you how to select appropriate types, tools, and designs for any evaluation and how to fit them into a structure that keeps an evaluation organized and on track. This kind of planning will enable you to efficiently provide clear information to management on program successes, failures, and opportunities.

The process of planning an evaluation can be organized into six steps:

1. Establish goals.
2. Identify evaluation resources.
3. Define the scope and specificity of evaluation by establishing appropriate dependent variables.
4. Decide on the design if one is required.
5. Determine how to measure the dependent variable, how to collect the data, and how the data will be analyzed.
6. Decide how the results will be reported.

The *General Evaluation Planning Checksheet* on page 136 is a form that you may copy to help you keep track of your progress as you proceed through the six steps of evaluation planning. Although this form also provides an overview of the evaluation planning process, you will not fully understand all the elements in it until you have completed this chapter.

The first two steps of evaluation planning—establishing goals and identifying resources—can be applied on two different levels, the macrolevel, and the microlevel. The macrolevel of steps one and two is what you do when you design an entire WHP program, including all the phases of evaluation that will be a part of it. This is the ideal way to approach planning because it means that you will be able to

- design each program and its evaluation to be part of an overall long-term plan to promote health and lower health care costs within your organization;
- plan all programs so that they lend themselves easily to evaluation;
- enlist the help and support (including financial) of decision makers in your company for an overall, effective WHP program as you plan; and
- take advantage of efficiencies within your company to share resources and goals not only among evaluation efforts but even among different departments and divisions of your company, thus maximizing the results of your evaluation dollars.

When you are planning evaluations on this scale, you will use the first two steps to establish your overall goals and identify evaluation resources for the master plan, enabling you to write a general outline of your organization's entire WHP program. Then you will plan each of the individual parts of the master plan one by one. This is the microlevel of planning, and it works best by far when it is done within the context of a WHP master plan. To do this, you will construct each separate intervention that is part of the master plan (see the author's text, *Worksite Health Promotion*, for a step-by-step approach to program planning), and you will design the assessments of each of those programs by applying all six steps listed above to each evaluation. You will repeat the process until you have designed all the individual parts of the master plan. As you work on each individual part, of course, you will be alert for indications that you have over- or underestimated the resources needed for various parts of the plan.

Therefore, you will need to make adjustments accordingly as you go, including getting the input of those who hold the purse strings of your organization. This sort of planning is usually done on an annual level when budgets are being set and other segments of the organization are also planning and making a bid for company resources. The *Planning Form for Goal Assessment* (page 137) is an example of a form that you might use on the microlevel of planning.

Unfortunately, you will find that in the real world of WHP promotion, you will often have to design the evaluation of a program without the benefit of an overall plan. This generally happens when you are brought into an organization

- that has an extremely small WHP program due to either the size of the establishment or its priorities;
- that has not had a WHP program before and has hired you in the middle of a fiscal year to start one;
- that has had a WHP program, but one that has never been planned on the macrolevel before: thus, for at least your first several months (and perhaps longer, depending on the political realities of your situation), you must work without the benefit of macrolevel planning; or
- that has called you in as a consultant to conduct an evaluation of a limited segment of its WHP program.

In all these situations, you will be unable to take advantage of the benefits of macro- or microlevel planning. You must simply start with setting evaluation goals for the assessment you have been asked to do, uncover whatever resources can be made available in a fiscal year that is already underway, and do the best you can with what you have as you proceed through steps two through six.

This chapter will discuss the first five of the six steps of WHP evaluation. The next chapter will include the sixth step, which is to decide how the results of evaluation will be reported. As the first five steps are described, remember that the first two (establishing goals and identifying evaluation resources) can be applied on either the macro- or microlevel. You will note that these levels are not differentiated in the text, but if you pay attention to the examples, you will be able to tell at which level the situation occurred. Noticing this will help you understand more clearly how to apply the principles discussed. And always remember, if feasible, apply goal setting and resource evaluation on a company-wide, long-term basis first, then design individual evaluations using steps one through six. It is the most effective approach to evaluation planning.

Step One: Establish Goals

To evaluate anything, of course, you have to know what it is you are evaluating. Thus, the first thing to do when planning an evaluation is to identify all those people who have a stake in knowing about the results of your proposed evaluation program and to find out what they are interested in knowing. Once you understand their interests, you can proceed with the task of developing appropriate evaluation goals. Before we proceed with how you do this, however, one caution: if you are either inexperienced or simply new to a company, it may be very useful to do a very quick, informal survey of possible available resources before developing goals. By doing so, you can get enough of a general idea of what resources are likely to be available to guide your goal planning. This should be very quick and will not take the place of the more detailed review of resources discussed in step two. Its function is merely to keep you from the extremes of grossly underestimating the possibilities or of being wildly optimistic about what can be done.

General Evaluation Planning Checksheet

	Measurable	Quantifiable	Achievable	Proposed time frame	Value to stakeholder
1. Establish evaluation goals					
•					
•					
•					

	On-site	Off-site	Availability	Cost
2. Identify evaluation resources				
• Personnel				
• Equipment				
• Materials				
• Facilities				
• Financial				

3. Define scope and specificity of evaluation

• Selected dependent variables (outcomes)

•

•

•

•

4. Decide on evaluation design, if one is required

_____

5. Plan for data analysis

A. How will dependent variable be measured?

B. How will data be analyzed?

C. Who will analyze data?

	In-person	E-mail	Hard copy	Meeting
6. How results will be reported				
• To management				
• To program staff				
• To employees				

From *Evaluating Worksite Health Promotion* by David H. Chenoweth, 2002, Champaign, IL: Human Kinetics.

Planning Form for Program Goal Assessment

Name of program: _____

Program goal being evaluated: _____

Program phase (check one): _____ pre-intervention _____ mid-intervention _____ post-intervention

Evaluation purpose: _____ program effectiveness _____ financial analysis

Ideal tool or design: _____

Quick estimate of resources needed (once you have listed what is needed, check those that are available):

1. Personnel: in-house vs. external?

_____

2. Equipment:

_____

3. Materials:

_____

4. Facilities:

_____

5. Time:

_____

6. Money:

_____

Realistic tool or design to be used: _____

Data management variable	Time frame, both length and intervals	Data needed, including source and measurement method	Who will measure and record
1.			
2.			
3.			
4.			

What Can You Do in 60 Days?

Suppose you recently joined the staff of a five-year-old worksite health promotion program which had never been formally evaluated. Staff members were recently told that the company is experiencing a tight cash-flow problem and is considering the elimination of several programs. Your boss, the human resources director, has informed the staff they must show that the program is worth its cost, or it will be on the chopping block. The program consists of a multifaceted array of health education seminars, a large state-of-the art fitness center, a work hardening facility, health screening services, an employee assistance program (EAP), and an on-site resource library. There's a sense of urgency in the air, as program continuation decisions will occur within 60 days. The worksite health promotion program director calls a staff meeting to discuss how to approach this challenging situation. Considering the broad scope of the program and the limited time frame available to demonstrate its value, one staff member suggests that a quick evaluation be done on whatever aspect of the overall program is believed to have the most impact on the company's bottom line. After further discussion, the staff unanimously selects the EAP for an evaluation on the premise that EAP services (a) probably have the highest benefit-to-cost ratio of any of the program offerings and (b) are viewed by management as an essential stress management resource for many employees working in an uncertain business climate. A quick assessment of evaluation resources is performed and reveals that in-house staff will have to do the evaluation because of a lack of time to secure a qualified off-site evaluator.

Identify Stakeholders

Designing an evaluation cannot be done effectively unless you include input from all the program stakeholders—those persons who have something to gain or lose from the evaluation results. Thus, you must establish who all the program stakeholders are and enlist their cooperation. Corporate financial officers, program administrators, health promotion staff members, program participants, and sponsors (if a funding source is involved) will probably all have questions they would like to have answered about the program. You will find that different stakeholders have different interests, and you must be sure to include evaluation goals that address all of their questions.

How can you be sure you have identified all the stakeholders? It will help if you will take four factors into account:

1. The administrative structure of an organization's key decision makers
2. The rationale for doing an evaluation
3. The history and maturity of the program being evaluated
4. The political realities surrounding the evaluation

Each of these four factors is important to consider. For example, a WHP director in a midsized company requested a claims data analysis from an outside vendor. The primary reason for doing the CDA was to establish a statistical baseline regarding the prevalence of employees' risk factors, so appropriate risk-reduction interventions could be established. Though she only requested that the report be directed to herself, the outside vendor proposed that it also be targeted to the human resource director and departmental representatives throughout the company. How did the four factors that can help you identify stakeholders affect this recommendation?

1. **The administrative structure of an organization's key decision makers:** Through discussions with the WHP director, the outside vendor discovered that she had requested that the vendor address several issues that had been identified by her

boss, the human resources director. Clearly, this person was a key decision maker in the WHP program.

2. **The rationale for doing the evaluation:** Since the evaluation initially centered on risk factor identification, the consultant recognized that the health management personnel who were responsible for creating and implementing specific risk-reduction programs should also receive the evaluation results.

3. **The history and maturity of the program being evaluated:** The vendor learned that the employee health promotion program was relatively new and that the WHP director was trying to expand it to reach a larger share of the workforce. This suggested to him that it was important to apprise departmental representatives of the program's current and future value, creating support throughout the company for the WHP director's intent.

4. **The political realities surrounding the evaluation:** The outside vendor learned from the WHP director that the human resources director and departmental heads had been influential in establishing past and present program policies. Thus, it was clear to him that without the support of the HR director and the department heads, the expansion of the program could not take place.

When the vendor shared his concerns about targeting the report to the HR director and the departmental heads as well as to the WHP director, she understood instantly that widening the audience for the report and addressing the concerns of the major stakeholders would significantly enhance her ability to push for the WHP program expansion.

Whose Business Is It Anyway?

The benefits director of a small West Coast medical center with approximately 250 employees hired an outside consulting company to conduct a review and cost-effectiveness comparison of its health care plan. She indicated that the analysis would be used by benefits personnel to determine if an outside managed care plan could offer a more competitive health care benefits package including on-site worksite health promotion programs for employees. The analysis was about to be submitted when the consulting firm learned from the benefits director that a new chief financial officer (CFO) had been hired and would be supervising all future benefits department activities. Because of this administrative change, the consultants quickly expanded the targeting of their recommendations to take into account the new CFO as a major stakeholder. If the benefits director had failed to notify the outside vendor of the administrative change, the new CFO would not have received essential data on the health plan options and, thus, not been in a position to consider vital financial criteria regarding worksite health promotion services decisions.

What kinds of questions will the stakeholders have? Program administrators may want to know if the operational expenses are within the designated budget; health promotion staff members may want to know if the incentives are motivating high-risk employees to participate; and funding sponsors may want to know if the money was spent wisely. The questions stakeholders will want answered will be as many and varied as the people involved. Finding out all of these questions may take some ingenuity. Based on an organization's culture and decision-making style, it may be appropriate to call a meeting of key decision makers. Another possibility may be to distribute a written survey or simply phone or e-mail them for feedback. In midsized and large companies, an annual worksite health promotion staff planning retreat may be held during which stakeholders are invited and asked to brainstorm with the staff on what programs and program evaluations they'd like to see in the future.

Health-Related Goals Versus Financial Goals

Goals of greatest interest to stakeholders are of two primary types: health-related and financial. If you fail to include both kinds of goals, you will also fail to plan for the evaluation types, designs, and instruments necessary to measure them.

Health-Related Goals

Evaluation will help determine whether health program goals and objectives are met, and it will also answer questions about the program as it is being implemented. Thus, evaluation planning should be closely tied to the development of an intervention's goals and objectives. If these goals and objectives are designed with ease of evaluation in mind, it can produce the following opportunities:

- Assessments can easily be made during the course of the program, enabling the organization to improve the program as it progresses. For example, if ongoing evaluations are scheduled, WHP personnel might discover that the low enrollment in a stress management workshop reflects an inadequate setting, inconvenient hours, or lack of publicity. These problems, once identified, could be addressed and eliminated.
- The clearly defined goals that evaluation requires can help program presenters and participants stay on track through ongoing mini-evaluations.

If the evaluation is not designed until the program has ended, neither of these benefits is possible. Moreover, carefully designed goals will enable you to focus on what the intervention can reasonably be expected to achieve, clarifying the impact of the intervention on its target.

The evaluation tools typically used to assess whether health-related goals have been achieved include claims data analysis and risk factor cost appraisal. These types of evaluation require data such as the total number of employees, percentage of employees with specific risk factors, and inpatient and outpatient claims data. Designs generally need to be selected and used to organize data collection during the intervention and to insure that it will be valid.

Financial Goals

Laudable as health-related goals may be, they cannot be pursued in isolation from financial goals. If money is not available to run the programs, the health-related goals will never be reached. Thus, it is crucial that health-related goals be attempted within the limitations imposed by financial necessity. These limitations will vary from organization to organization, depending on the financial resources of those organizations as well as on the values of those who control the purse strings.

Key decision makers who hold the purse strings are usually interested in financial goals. They will want to ask questions that can be answered by using evaluation instruments such as break-even analysis, cost-effectiveness analysis, forecasting, and benefit-cost analysis. Standard data needed for these evaluations include programming costs (fixed and variable), outcomes, participation rates, length of intervention, and the nature of significant trends.

Goal Criteria

Because you are developing your evaluation goals in connection with specific programs, you must think not only about goals that are exclusively concerned with evaluation but about the general goals of the WHP programs as well. If the goals of those programs are intelligently developed, it will make your evaluation goals that much easier to develop. Evaluation is greatly enhanced when the program being evaluated contains goals that are developed according to the following five criteria:

1. **Compatibility with stakeholders' personal health or values**—The desirable outcome is valued by participants, program personnel, top management, or other stakeholders.

2. **Quantifiability**—Evaluators can track and attach a statistical value (#, $, %) to the dependent variable.

3. **Measurability**—Evaluators can physically record changes that may occur in the outcome (dependent) variable and can do so in a manner that is statistically significant.

4. **Sufficient intervention time frame**—The intervention will be offered for an amount of time believed necessary to see a favorable impact.

5. **Realistic achievability**—There is strong likelihood the intervention will favorably impact the dependent variable.

It is not uncommon to see organizational health promotion goals that lack one or more of the five criteria. An example of such a goal would be, *Within one year, workers' compensation costs will decrease by at least 20%.* Here, in contrast, is a goal that incorporates all five criteria: *Within six months* [time frame], *60%* [realistically achievable] *of the male employee population* [stakeholders] *will have blood pressures of 130-85 or less* [quantifiable] *as measured at their annual physical exam* [measurability].

Defining a Goal You Can Handle

Suppose one of the goals of your low back injury prevention program is, *Reduce absenteeism by 20% within six months.* Stated as such, the goal implies all absences regardless of their cause. Yet, is it realistic to expect that the low back injury prevention program can affect all absences? Probably not, because many absences are not due to low back injuries or, for that matter, any other health status indicator. In fact, many absences are due to uncontrollable and unanticipated events such as serving on jury duty, picking up a sick child from school, attending a funeral, and work dissatisfaction. Based on this qualification, a more appropriate goal of the low back injury prevention program would be, *Reduce absenteeism exclusively due to low back pain or injury by 20% within six months.* Note that the clause *exclusively due to low back pain or injury* defines the scope and specificity of the goal.

Let's take a couple of goals that are not very useful for either planning or evaluation and, by applying the five goal criteria, rewrite them until they are useful for evaluation. Suppose that your two goals are the following:

- Improve the cardiovascular health of female employees.
- Improve employee productivity.

Now, one by one, here is how adding the elements defined in each of the criteria can transform these valueless goals into valuable tools for planning both programs and evaluation:

1. **Compatibility with stakeholders' personal health or values.** When you are creating your goals, you must be certain that they will be supported by the stakeholders. Say, for example, that after you decided on your goals, you ran a survey on the 400 women in your workforce and learned that the primary health concern of 350 of them was breast cancer. In that case, you would have a hard time selling your cardiovascular endurance program. If you had limited funds and could afford only one major program for women, you would want to change the focus of your goal. You might begin to rewrite it as, *Reduce personal risk of breast cancer for female employees.* Of course, you would have saved yourself some trouble had you surveyed the stakeholders in your women's health program before you decided on your goal. We will assume that you had surveyed major stakeholders already about employee productivity; thus, that goal will remain the same.

2. **Quantifiability.** Although both of your goals are now compatible with the interests of your stakeholders, neither is particularly useful yet because neither contains anything that can be quantified. One way of stating this requirement for quantifiability would be to say that in order for a goal statement to be measurable, it must contain a dependent variable. To review material from chapter 2, a dependent variable is an observable property that varies—that is, takes on different values, depending on the impact of the intervention (independent variable)—and to which numbers can be assigned. Examples of dependent variables would be blood pressure, sick-leave absenteeism, medical claim costs, and productivity. Establishing valid dependent variables is discussed at length on pages 14-25. The unsatisfactory goals above can be redeemed by assigning each of them a quantifiable variable factor (dependent variable) that could serve as a measurement of progress toward the general goal. Consider the following as examples:

- Reduce personal risk of breast cancer for female employees *as shown by at least a 50% reduction in risk factor prevalence for breast cancer in the female workforce.*
- Improve employee productivity through a *reduction in on-the-job tardiness and absenteeism of at least 30%.*

You can see that the second version of each goal includes a measurable factor. You can also see from the two examples that it is not possible to write measurable program goals in the absence of baseline data. You cannot, after all, tell when an improvement in anything has occurred if you do not know what the original level was. Thus, if there is no baseline for the area being measured, the first goal should be to establish one. For our goals, for example, one would first need to know the current breast cancer risk factor status of the female workforce. Second, data about absenteeism are needed— something like the average tardiness rate per six months and average absenteeism rate per six months for the last three years. In the case of certain program evaluation goals, the baseline could be established in the first evaluation time frame.

3. **Measurability.** Now that you have quantified your goals, your next step is to be sure that you have the means to measure them. Continuing with our example, you must ask yourself what resources are available for measuring breast cancer risk, on-the-job tardiness, and absenteeism. For example, will breast cancer risk be assessed via personalized HRAs, self-reported feedback, clinical screening, or medical claims data? Do supervisors have the proper tools to easily monitor tardiness and absenteeism? It is crucial that you secure the proper personnel and equipment for monitoring the measurable factors of your goals before you proceed with your evaluation.

4. **Sufficient intervention time frame.** In order to know how to plan and how to evaluate, you must also include some kind of time frame in your goals. Consider these examples:

- Improve the health of female employees as shown by at least a 50% reduction in risk factor prevalence for breast cancer in the female workforce *within six months.*
- Improve employee productivity through a reduction in on-the-job tardiness and absenteeism of at least 30% *in four months.*

Now you have a defined target at which you can aim. Without a definite deadline to aim for, your measurement of progress would not be very meaningful. Only if you know how you're doing within a time frame can you know whether you need to change your tactics to be more effective or whether it would be reasonable to set your sights higher than your original goal.

5. **Realistic achievability.** It is important to establish a goal that is realistically achievable in order not to create false expectations for yourself or others. Although the goals developed so far are compatible with stakeholders' personal goals and feature both measurability and chronological definition, you must also be sure that they are realistic. How do you do this? You can form a good idea of what is realistic in your situation by studying similar programs and learning what their results have been, as well as the factors that have affected their success rates. In doing so, you should look for significant differences between your situation and those of the programs studied—for example, differences in education level, age of participants, and geographic differences (i.e., smoking reduction might not be as successful in tobacco-growing areas as in silicon valley). Consulting an expert is also a useful strategy. Once you do your homework regarding the two goals we have been developing, you discover that, in fact, they are not realistic. Based on what you have learned, then, the revisions you make to your goals are as follows:

- Improve the health of female employees as evidenced by at least a 25% reduction in risk factor prevalence for breast cancer in the female workforce *within one year.*
- Improve employee productivity through a reduction in on-the-job tardiness and absenteeism of at least 10% *in six months.*

Some evaluation experts recommend that once you establish what seem to be objective goals, you lower your sights a few percentage points to take into account differences you may have overlooked. If you have a general idea of what you'd like to accomplish in your WHP program, applying this five-goal criteria to those general ideas will yield goals that are quantifiable, measurable, realistic, chronologically defined, and compatible with your stakeholders' interests. Such goals are indispensable for valid evaluation as well as for program development.

Establishing Measurable Objectives

Once program goals have been developed, it is time to establish measurable objectives to indicate what actions must be undertaken to attain each goal. Objectives are stepping stones, or rungs on a ladder, that enable program planners to achieve a particular goal. As an evaluator, you should be very interested in objectives because properly written objectives will facilitate and enhance the quality of the evaluation process and results.

When constructing objectives you should do the following:

- Establish short-term objectives to use in monitoring progress in the initial phase of the intervention—for example, *At the end of one month, at least 75% of all original participants will be actively involved in personalized risk-reduction programs.*

- Establish long-range objectives to determine if initial levels of progress have been sustained—for example, *At the end of six months, at least 50% of all participants achieving initial risk-reduction goals will have maintained or exceeded that level of success.*

- Avoid the temptation to establish a long list of objectives, especially if the intervention to be evaluated is short-term, if evaluations have not been conducted in the past, or if an evaluation will be used as a prelude to a more formalized and thorough evaluation. Too many objectives can add unnecessary procedures that will increase the costs of conducting an evaluation.

- Include objectives that identify specific resources needed to achieve the goal—for example, *Develop a health care provider network of personal physicians for at-risk referrals.*

- Specify time frames when appropriate—for example, *All participants will be screened at a minimum on a quarterly basis and more frequently if they are classified as high-risk.*

Properly written objectives are invaluable in planning the evaluation process. Suppose, for example, that the primary goal of a prenatal health enhancement program at a large manufacturing site (900 employees) is, *Increase the percentage of healthy babies at least 20% for employees and dependents within 12 months.* Sample objectives associated with this goal follow. You can see that if all of the objectives are achieved, the goal with which they are associated will have been reached. Note that some of these objectives are not directly related to evaluation (e.g., *Initiate on-site programs and additional referrals . . .*), yet the programs required by the objectives (i.e., the effectiveness of the on-site and additional referral program) will need to be evaluated. You must plan for those evaluations at this stage. The program objectives tell you what data you will need to collect, how often you will need to analyze it, and what instruments you will need to use. Each goal objective below is followed by appropriate evaluation planning decisions you may make based on that objective.

- **Objective 1:** Identify population at risk—all female employees and dependents who incurred a pregnancy complication in the past two years. **Evaluation planning decisions:** During weeks 1-4, contact insurer or TPA to obtain medical claims data on the number of all pregnancy complications.

- **Objective 2:** Conduct an analysis of pregnancy claims data from the past two years to identify specific types of pregnancy-related complications. Review specific complications by ICD and DRG. **Evaluation planning decisions:** During weeks 5-6, develop a framework in which to record the number of each type of complication that has occurred in the past two years.

- **Objective 3:** Develop an expanded prenatal screening and health education program with financial incentives. **Evaluation planning decisions:** During weeks 7-8, develop a framework to track participation in the screening and program.

- **Objective 4:** Inform all women of the new program and incentives via bulletin boards, paycheck stuffers, e-mails, and newsletters. **Evaluation planning decisions:** During weeks 9-10, prepare a format to list distribution activities.

- **Objective 5:** Provide orientation sessions including a comprehensive health screening to identify women at risk of pregnancy complications; construct a format for collecting baseline data. **Evaluation planning decisions:** During weeks 11-12, establish a two-group, quasi-experimental evaluation design.

- **Objective 6:** Initiate on-site programs and additional referrals to personal physicians for selected women, if necessary. **Evaluation planning decisions:** During weeks 13-18, record the names and numbers of on-site participants and off-site referrals.

- **Objective 7:** Monitor health status of at-risk women at appropriate (risk-based) intervals. Provide customized interventions for each woman. **Evaluation planning decisions:** During weeks 24 and 30, compare baseline health status levels versus 6 months and 12 months levels. Analyze interval-to-interval changes to determine the intervention impact.

One Approach to Developing Program Objectives

One way to develop program objectives is to think about the items within the goal that you want to evaluate, then restate them as tasks rather than objectives. For example, your goal is, *Reduce the direct cost of low back injuries to the company's warehouse and shipping workforce by 20% within 18 months.* You come up with the following items to be evaluated:

- Total medical claims for low back injuries
- Total participation as a percentage of the eligible population
- Total number of departmental supervisors who qualify for bonuses, based on program participation or enhanced productivity by their employees
- Total number of injury-free work hours by program participants

Based on this list of items, your program objectives would be as follows:

1. Conduct an analysis of medical claims for low back injuries in the warehouse and shipping workforce to identify the most common causes of injury.
2. Develop a low back injury prevention program based on results of medical claims analysis.
3. Develop an incentive program for participation—include incentives for both workers and supervisors.
4. Measure program participation.
5. Measure changes in workforce productivity.
6. Compare total number of injury-free work hours by program participants and nonparticipants.

REVIEW QUESTIONS: GENERAL PLANNING AND DEVELOPING GOALS

1. Upon reviewing the staff's course of action in *Design Deliberations* (page 157), decide whether the selected strategy represented macrolevel planning, microlevel planning, or some of both. Justify your answer. Look at *What Can You Do in 60 Days?* (page 138) and *One Approach to Developing Program Objectives* (above), and answer the same question.
2. Who are the major stakeholders to consider in a program evaluation?
3. When and why is it important to distinguish between health-related goals and financial goals?
4. What are the major criteria that an evaluation goal should meet? Discuss each one.
5. Choose any program goal from this book and develop objectives for it that lend themselves to unambiguous evaluation.

Step Two: Identify Evaluation Resources

Some of those who evaluate organizational health interventions worry that their evaluation efforts do not meet the requirements of traditional social science research. Research requires rigorous controls, strict isolation of program elements, and long-term follow-up. On the contrary, implementation and evaluation of worksite health promotion interventions generally must be done with limitations on time, personnel, finances, data availability, and conflicting organizational needs that make meeting the demands of research impossible. The evaluator, rather than feeling frustrated, must realize that evaluation is not research and therefore does not require the same resources or strict controls. Evaluation is a step that is taken to improve a program; research is done to validate a hypothesis. In all likelihood the resources and requirements of your organizational setting will not allow rigorous research: You must simply assess your resources and devise the best possible evaluation program possible with whatever means you are able to find within the organization.

The following are resources you should consider as you begin planning evaluations:

- **Financial resources.** During budget-cutting times, financial resources may be limited. In those instances, it is important to identify alternative sources of funding as well as how to use other resources creatively to lessen the need for money. For example, consider approaching your insurer or managed care provider to see if they would be willing to fund a portion of an evaluation project. This could be proposed on the premise that the evaluation could demonstrate their commitment toward enhancing your efforts to improve employees' health and contain health care costs. A second strategy is to contact a local university to see if a professor could assist you with an evaluation in exchange for having for a worksite to conduct some research. Another option is to explore with the local health department or state health department whether any grants are available through their offices that could be applied toward a program evaluation. Finally, professional organizations often have a member who may be willing to provide an on-site evaluation at a discounted price with the promise of business in the future, provided that you like the evaluator's work.

- **Personnel.** You should assess how much staff is available to you and what skills they possess. If the available skill level is low, you should think about how to adjust your expectations and methods, how to arrange for additional training, or how to find outside resources who can help you. The principles discussed in detail in chapter 3 on how to find an outside firm to do CDA can be adapted to searching for outside resources for other purposes as well.

- **Equipment and materials.** Although a minimum of two measurements (baseline and outcome) are typical in most evaluations, projects involving multiple measurements (such as those in time series designs) may require additional resources to complete the full evaluation. For instance, if most of the employee participants in an on-site exercise program are expected to record their daily workouts on a specific computer program to be used for future research, adequate time and computer resources should be arranged to ensure a smooth data entry operation.

- **Facilities.** Program evaluation involves various daily tasks that require a clean, organized setting. Some evaluations involve personal and confidential data that should be housed in a protective setting away from the mainstream of unauthorized personnel. Therefore, to ensure a suitable environment for quality evaluation, evaluators may need to secure a safe location to store and analyze evaluation resources and data.

- **Schedule.** Evaluation planning involves scheduling considerations for those doing the evaluation and for those being evaluated. The latter is particularly important in worksites operating on assembly-line manufacturing schedules or similar

Evaluation Resource Assessment Grid for One Goal

Goal: _____

Objectives	Funding	Personnel	Equipment	Facilities
1.				
2.				
3.				
4.				
5.				
6.				

arrangements in which there is little or no flextime for employees. By considering employees' workshifts and workloads, evaluations can be arranged to accommodate the schedules of all stakeholders.

A sample resource assessment grid is shown on page 147. You may copy or adapt this grid for use in planning evaluations. Note that the grid is formatted for only one goal. In the event that an evaluation contains several goals (which is usually the case), keep all the goals for that evaluation in a folder, or staple all the goals for the evaluation together.

Step Three: Define Scope and Specificity

The structure of your evaluation is influenced largely by the scope and specificity of your evaluation needs. **Scope** refers to the range of variables and the time frame of the evaluation. For example, an evaluation consisting of several variables that are measured over a one-year time frame has a broader scope than an evaluation involving one or two variables spanning a period of six months. In contrast, **specificity** refers to the level or degree of precision evaluators use in measuring selected variables within an evaluation.

Establishing the Scope of Your Evaluation

The scope of your evaluation will be defined by the number of variables you choose to look at and the time frame in which you do so. For example, the scope of a back injury prevention program evaluation will probably be smaller than a medical self-care program evaluation. The back program evaluation is more likely to focus on a single variable (number of back injuries) that can be influenced in a relatively short time frame, whereas the medical self-care program is likely to include multiple variables (e.g., health care claims and health care costs) that usually take longer to be influenced by the intervention.

Determining an Appropriate Range of Variables

Use these questions to determine which variables may be most appropriate in a specific evaluation:

- What variables are believed to be of greatest value to stakeholders?
- Which variables can be tracked and quantified?
- Which variables are likely to be influenced in a short period of time? In a longer time frame?
- How much time is management giving program providers to show results? (See table 5.1 for variables that can be affected in short time frames.)
- Which variables may require financial resources to evaluate beyond what is currently available?

When deciding what dependent variables to evaluate, keep in mind that some decision makers prefer to look at absolute numbers while other decision makers prefer relative numbers, such as rates per employee or cost as a percentage of income. Examples of variables based on **absolute numbers** are

- number of health care claims incurred by employees,
- health care costs paid by an organization,

Table 5.1 Outcome Variables That Can Be Affected by Short-Term Interventions

Intervention	Outcome variable affected	
Back injury prevention	• Absences • Health care usage	• Health care costs • Productivity
Cardiac rehabilitation	• Absences • Health care costs	• Return-to-work time frame
Diabetes education/control	• Absences • Health care usage • Health care costs	• Hypoglycemia • Diabetes complications
Drug abuse treatment	• Accidents and injuries • Health care costs • Malnutrition	• Over-dependence on health care system • Seizures
Exercise	• Absences • Anxiety • Blood pressure • Depression • Diabetes Type II • Health care costs • Health care usage	• Job satisfaction • Morale • Musculoskeletal conditions • Obesity • Productivity • Turnover
Immunizations	• Hepatitis • Influenza (flu)	• Pneumonia • Tetanus
Medical self-care	• Diagnostic testing • Elective surgery • Health care usage	• Health care costs • Prescription medication usage • Over-the-counter medication usage
Safety education/incentives	• Absences • Accidents/injuries • Health care costs	• Health care usage • Productivity
Seat belt safety	• Health care costs • Health care usage	• Motor vehicle accident-induced trauma
Smoking cessation	• Absences • Asthma • Bronchitis • Upper-respiratory infections	• Health care usage • Health care costs • Pregnancy outcomes for mother and baby • Upper-respiratory infections

- total number of workers' compensation claims,
- average length of stay for all DRGs.

Examples of **rate-based variables** include
- cost of medical benefits spent per employee,
- volume of medical care services used per family,
- price of medical services used to treat a specific risk factor,
- disability payments per employee.

If you have determined that your stakeholders have preferences about absolute versus rate-based variables, you must be sure to make this distinction and select your variables accordingly.

What Are You Looking At?

A large beverage manufacturer called in a consultant to evaluate its multifaceted health promotion program. The program was nationally known for its state-of-the-art fitness center, on-site cardiac rehabilitation program, employee-oriented health education seminars, and participation-based financial incentives. Several years earlier the company had hired a local consultant to do a benefit-cost analysis (BCA) on the entire program. The BCA yielded a benefit-cost ratio of 75 cents to the dollar, or a loss of 25 cents per programming dollar. The BCA study was shared with the second consultant before his on-site visit to familiarize him with that evaluation's methodology, outcome variables, and results. The BCA study focused on two outcome variables:

1. Organizational health care costs

2. On-the-job accidents

Moreover, the consultant noticed that baseline (pre-intervention) levels for both variables were actually lower than the industry norm and the national norm and that the evaluation time frame of six months was very short considering the nature of both outcome variables. Thus he was not surprised to see the less than favorable benefit-cost ratio.

When the new consultant made an on-site visit, he indicated to health management staff members that the original evaluation may have been misleading because

- variable #1 was too generically defined;
- variable #2 did not reflect the full scope of the multifaceted program;
- the baseline levels for both variables were too low; and
- the evaluation time frame was too short for programmatic interventions to significantly influence the outcome variables.

The consultant indicated that the proposed program evaluation could avoid the preceding pitfalls with proper planning and input from all stakeholders. First, he asked staff members to identify a list of key outcome variables pertinent to their individual departments. Staff members identified 15 outcome variables ranging from absenteeism to workers' compensation costs. The consultant then facilitated a discussion on which of the outcome measures met key selection criteria, such as measurability, quantifiability, and relevance. This process guided all parties to design the new evaluation in which

- several variables were selected that reflected the scope of the program;
- variables selected had baseline readings at or above the industry and national norms;
- each of the selected variables was narrowly defined (e.g., health care costs related to back injuries); and
- a one-year evaluation time frame was selected to provide adequate time for interventions to make an impact.

With the preceding revisions in place, a new evaluation was done, and it provided the organization with a more objective analysis of its entire program.

Determining an Appropriate Time Frame

The other aspect of evaluation scope is its time frame. Have you ever heard the saying, *Timing is everything*? It certainly applies to program evaluation. Program evaluation timing questions include the following:

- What period should an evaluation cover?
- When should measurements be taken?
- How often should wide-scale evaluations be conducted?

The answer to each of these issues depends, in part, on an organization's resources and experience.

What Period Should an Evaluation Cover?

Organizations with little evaluation experience may benefit initially by doing a short-term evaluation in which they can become familiar with the evaluation process and learn from initial mistakes before proceeding to a comprehensive, long-term evaluation. Short-term evaluations are particularly suitable with the following circumstances:

- The intervention includes only a small number of participants.
- There is a strong likelihood of employee turnover or absenteeism, the effects of which will be magnified by length of time.
- The intervention can be offered only for a short period of time.
- Financial resources are limited.
- Key decision makers are skeptical about the value of the intervention.
- Evaluation personnel are available only for a short period of time.
- Access to retrospective (historical) data is limited.
- The intervention is likely to make a measurable impact on the dependent variable in a short time.

Of course, there are many factors that influence the amount of time it takes for an intervention to have a measurable impact, including the level of participants' interest, availability of incentives, time of the intervention, and the personality of the instructor. Many variables are by nature better suited to some time frames than others. Some examples follow:

- **Short-term time frame (1-6 months)**
  - Accidents/injuries
  - Attitude/morale (job satisfaction)
  - Health care utilization (emergency department visits)
  - Risk factor status indicators (blood pressure, blood glucose, physical activity, tobacco use, etc.)
- **Intermediate time frame (6-12 months)**
  - Absenteeism
  - Case management of chronic ailments (diabetes, heart disease, etc.)
  - Health care utilization (overall)
  - Risk factor status indicators (serum cholesterol, illegal drug use)
  - Productivity
  - Workers' compensation claims
- **Long-term time frame (> 1 year)**
  - Health care charges (specific)
  - Workers' compensation charges

In establishing an appropriate time frame for an evaluation, it is important to consider some of the advantages and limitations inherent in each option (see table 5.2) and how these interact with the program evaluation timing questions listed at the beginning of this section. For example, a short-term time frame may be more suitable in settings with limited finances, low number of participants, no control or comparison group, or little need to do an extensive evaluation. In contrast, results generated in an intermediate evaluation carry more credibility than a short-term impact. Finally, while a long-term evaluation may require more teamwork and financial resources, it is more accommodating to the econometric analyses highlighted in chapter 4.

When Should Measurements Be Taken?

To create a successful evaluation strategy, it is important to anticipate what, if any, periodic evaluations (and hence, measurements) should occur during a particular intervention. A short-term goal may call for weekly or monthly data measurements for process and impact evaluation, whereas a long-term goal may warrant quarterly or semiannual measurements for outcome evaluation. It is often true that an intervention will contain not one, but several goals, and that some of these will be long-term while others will be short-term. Whether an intervention or evaluation has (a) one goal or many goals or (b) all short-term, all long-term, or mixed goals, you must specify what data are needed for each goal and when. Construct a schedule for

Table 5.2 Advantages and Limitations Associated With Specific Evaluation Time Frames

Time frame	Potential advantages	Potential limitations
Short-term (1-6 months)	Inexpensive; can usually be conducted by 1-2 evaluators	Hawthorne or sentinel effect can be the primary influence on dependent variable
	Suitable for a pilot study	Insufficient time to recruit and influence hard-to-reach individuals
	Opportunity to identify and learn from mistakes for future evaluation	Low probability for doing econometric analyses (e.g., break-even, cost-effectiveness, benefit-cost, forecasting)
Intermediate (6-12 months)	Can modify intervention if the initial version is not working	May require extra personnel to evaluate if original plans are not sound
	Results carry more credibility than short-term	Feasibility of doing a multiyear forecast is questionable
	Cost-effectiveness analysis is usually feasible if two or more similar interventions are underway for a similar time frame	Uncertainty exists if any changes occurring near the end of this phase are by chance and likely to be sustained
	Break-even analysis is feasible if benefits are accruing within time of intervention	
Long-term (> 1 year)	Additional modifications to interventions may be possible	Can be costly, especially if evaluation lingers on without a set end line
	More time to recruit hard-to-reach individuals	Requires more teamwork and coordination among and between all parties
	Results carry high credibility	
	More opportunity to do econometric analysis	

appropriate measurement and recording of each of the goals throughout the duration of the intervention being evaluated. Figure 5.1 is an example of a schedule that clearly delineates what is to be measured and when it is to be measured. For every evaluation that you plan, you should create such a framework to guide evaluators and program staff through this important process. It will also be useful to make a chart similar to the one in the *Planning Form for Program Goal Assessment* on page 137 and to fill in the information asked for in that form regarding by whom, where, and how the measurements will be done. By filling out and keeping these tools together and accessible to the staff, you can ensure that everyone will be clear on the procedures. Of course, if your staff is small, virtually all of the tasks will be done by one or two people. In that case, it will not be essential to factor in the *by whom* dimension.

How Often Should Wide-Scale Evaluations Be Conducted?

Wide-scale evaluations involving outcome variables such as absenteeism, health care utilization, and health care costs are usually done over a long-term time frame because these variables are difficult to influence in the short-term. Moreover, establishing baseline and interval measurements on these types of variables generally requires the efforts of several health management personnel who must be able to identify and procure specific data from their databases. Coordinating their efforts would be more time consuming than could be justified in an evaluation with a short time frame.

Establishing the Specificity of Your Evaluation

Specificity refers to the degree of precision used by evaluators in defining outcome variables. For example, an outcome variable such as *absenteeism* has virtually no level

	Time frame						
Short-term goals	Baseline	2 mos	4 mos	6 mos	8 mos	10 mos	12 mos
• Increase the **number of employees practicing safe lifting procedures**							
• Reduce the **number of on-the-job back injuries**							
Long-term goals	Baseline	6 mos		12 mos		18 mos	24 mos
• Reduce **low back injury costs**							
• Reduce **low-back injury-related absences**							
• Increase **production output** in selected departments at highest risk of back injuries							

Figure 5.1   Sample schedule for taking measurements in a complex intervention.

of specificity because it does not delineate specific types (reasons for) of absenteeism. In contrast, an outcome variable such as *absenteeism due to low back injuries* has some level of specificity because it specifies the context of absenteeism. Programs that include outcome variables with a high level of specificity are preferred because they provide evaluators with greater opportunities to closely study the real impact of an intervention on a particular variable. For example

Variable	Less specificity	More specificity
• Absenteeism	(all causes)	Due to sick leave
• Health care claims	Total number	Number by type of claim
• Participation	Per month	Per week
• High-risk employees	Total number	Number by age and gender
• Injuries	Total number	Number incurred on the job

Defining highly specific variables is only possible if problems and needs are carefully analyzed. *Simplify!* provides an excellent example of how one company wrote a dependent variable with a high degree of specificity based on a careful examination of the wide range of factors affecting their rising health care costs.

Simplify!

A midsized West Coast utility company had been experiencing double-digit health care cost inflation over the past few years. Health management staff members reviewed several years of claims data and noticed that emergency department (ED) utilization was the fastest-growing claim during this time frame and that 35- to 45-year-old women had the highest ED usage, followed closely by 25- to 35-year-old men. The identified group of women worked primarily in the customer service department while the targeted males worked in the line repair division. Small group sessions with both groups were conducted to identify what factors were causing higher ED usage among these particular groups. Both groups indicated similar reasons for their ED usage: Many customer complaints reported in the late afternoon required customer service representatives to stay beyond their scheduled 5 P.M. quitting time and thus prevented them from seeking care from their managed care providers; and many line repairmen used the ED because they often worked overtime because of late-afternoon power failures. A final review of individual ED claims by the occupational health nurse indicated that virtually all of the health problems prompting ED visits were not emergencies, but minor ailments such as colds, sore muscles, and skin rashes. Realizing they could do little to influence the timing of customer complaints and power shortages, health management personnel decided to try reducing ED utilization by teaching and motivating employees to treat minor ailments through a medical self-care (MSC) program. The health management staff established a program goal of *reducing the number of ED visits associated with minor ailments by 25% within one year,* based on a review of MSC program results reported in the professional literature. The MSC program included weekly small-group seminars during an expanded lunch period. By taking into consideration each target group's work schedule and health problems, health management staff were able to establish a manageable **scope** (selecting the fastest-growing claim, allowing ample time for the program to have an effect before evaluating it) and **specificity** (zeroing in on only nonemergency ailments) for the program dependent variables, ensuring among other things that the program could be easily evaluated.

> ## REVIEW QUESTIONS: RESOURCES AND SCOPE AND SPECIFICITY
>
> 1. Differentiate between research and evaluation.
> 2. Discuss the six types of resources you must consider as you plan WHP evaluation.
> 3. Why is it important to consider the background of staff members before assigning evaluation duties?
> 4. How do you establish the scope of an evaluation?
> 5. How do you establish the specificity of an evaluation?

Step Four: Select an Evaluation Design

As you may recall from chapter 2, not all evaluations require a design—only program effectiveness evaluations do. Evaluation designs vary greatly by their type, scope, specificity, and feasibility. In deciding which evaluation design to select, evaluators should consider each of the following questions:

- What is the purpose (goal) of the evaluation?
- How much control do evaluators have over what groups are selected?
- Who will receive a specific intervention?
- Are there opportunities for matching a comparison group with the experimental group?
- What outcome variables will be evaluated? For how long?
- Are resources available for one or two measurements or for multiple measurements?
- Is the planned evaluation suited more toward quantitative data, qualitative data, or both?

These questions are important guideposts to use in narrowing the choice of evaluation designs. Here are more specific factors to consider in the areas of evaluation purpose and resources:

- **Purpose of the evaluation.** Some designs are better than others for particular purposes. Consider the following examples:

  - If you wish to measure the impact of a short-term intervention, say, on a pilot basis, a simple one group pre- and post-test design will usually be sufficient.
  - If you want more rigor in your evaluation, you may opt to compare participants against a matched group of nonparticipants.
  - If you need to compare two versions of an intervention, a good option is a quasi-experimental design in which the self-selected employees are randomly assigned to each option.
  - If your question is whether timing (e.g., a particular season) and associated events had an additional influence beyond the intervention, a staggered evaluation design would be most appropriate.
  - If you want to minimize the impact of any interval-to-interval group differences on the outcome variable, you could use a multiple time series design.
  - If you intend to publish your research in a professional, peer-reviewed article, you should choose either a true experimental or quasi-experimental design. You can only make this last choice, of course, if you have sufficient resources available to you.

Table 5.3 Sample Goals With Appropriate Designs and Tools

	Phase 1 preintervention	Phase 2 midintervention	Phase 3 postintervention
Goal	To establish a baseline prescription	To determine if an intervention is progressing as expected	To determine if an intervention has made a favorable impact
Design options: Time series; pre- and post-test; staggered; post-test only			
Goal	To identify health care use and cost trends	To determine which intervention *may* produce the best value	To project probable outcomes
Tools	Claims data analysis	Cost-effectiveness analysis	Forecast
Goal	To calculate the cost of risk factors	To determine if, and when, projected benefits will equal costs	To compare benefits vs. costs
Tools	Risk factor cost appraisal	Break-even analysis	Benefit-cost analysis

Table 5.3 illustrates typical designs and tools used in connection with specific goals during each phase of an intervention.

- **Evaluation resources.** Evaluation resources can either limit your design resources or open them up. Many worksite health management personnel would prefer to use true experimental designs for their program evaluation. However, given the personnel and the ethical, financial, and scheduling realities facing most worksite settings, true experimental designs are usually not possible. If that is the case in your own situation, you should next consider quasi-experimental designs. If your resources will not permit quasi-experimental designs either, you will most likely have to settle for nonexperimental designs, which are the least powerful option. If, however, you plan the evaluations involving nonexperimental designs carefully and work hard to note all external factors that could possibly be influencing the dependent variables, you can still arrive at reasonably reliable conclusions. Here are some specific resource considerations for various designs:

  - Time series and long-term designs generally require more resources than pretest–post-test designs and short-term designs because of the increased number of measurements and personnel needed.

  - If a measuring instrument has only one version, evaluators will generally restrict its use to no more than a pretest–post-test format to minimize testing and other threats to internal validity (see chapter 2).

  - If evaluators can be retained for a lengthy period of time, a multigroup design is more feasible than if you are having to rely on outside consultants and if you have a limited budget to spend on them.

  - If financial resources are severely limited, you will almost always have to use only a short-term, pretest–post-test design.

Figure 5.2 summarizes how both resources and other factors will be affected by your choice of benefits to assess.

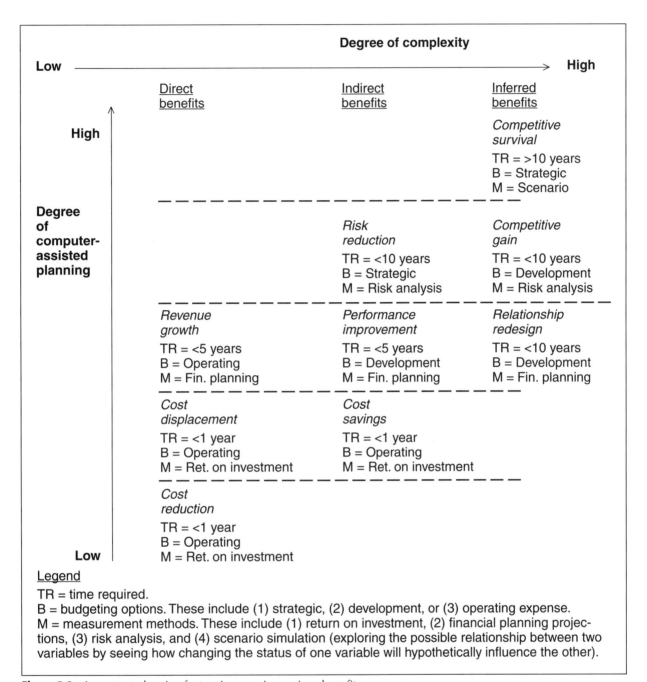

Figure 5.2 Important planning factors in assessing various benefits.

■ **Design Deliberations**

A northern U.S. grain processing company with nearly 1,000 employees wanted to evaluate the impact of a prework, back-stretching program on the annual prevalence and cost of low back injuries. Despite its size, the organization had only one full-time health management staff member—an occupational health nurse—who decided to relegate the bulk of the evaluation to an independent health management consultant.

(continued)

(continued)

The consultant and the nurse decided that the goal of the evaluation would be to determine if a five-minute, prework, back-stretching routine could reduce the prevalence and average cost of on-the-job, low back injuries. Considerations—both ethical (they didn't want to deny chances for improved health to any worker) and statistical (the greater the proportion of participants, the more significant any changes evident at the end of the evaluation program would be)—required that they find a way to motivate as many employees as possible to participate in the daily, five-minute intervention. To achieve this goal, management offered employees a strong financial incentive: *Employees who participate in at least 90% of all prework stretch sessions will equitably share 50% of any cost-savings resulting from the intervention.* The incentive attracted 75% of all employees, including all but two employees in the three departments judged to have the highest risk of back injury.

By using a simple one-group, pretest–post-test design, they could have determined pretty clearly whether the intervention had an effect at the end of the evaluation period. The consultant, however, pointed out that for very little extra money, a quasi-experimental two-group comparison group design could be used, enabling them to also tell which of two different interventions was the more effective. The participants would be randomly assigned to a low back stretch routine designed by the occupational health nurse or to a similar routine recommended by a local group of physical therapists. By assigning participants to either of the two options, the evaluation design enabled the company not only to tell whether the stretching routine would improve the health of the employees and the company's bottom line, but also to compare both stretching routines head-to-head.

Step Five: Manage Data

There are three essential tasks involving data that must be done if evaluation is to be successful. These are

- acquiring and monitoring data, which involves getting existing data from in-house and out-of-house sources, and arranging for the gathering and recording future data, both in-house and out-of-house;
- analyzing data, which has been discussed at length in chapters 3 and 4; and
- reporting data, which is discussed in chapter 6.

Three things must be kept in mind as you plan evaluation data management:

1. The goals of your WHP programs that must be evaluated
2. The questions that must be answered to evaluate those goals (these questions can generally be generated from the objectives for each goal)
3. The answers to the what-who-where-how-when questions—sometimes called *Socratic elements*, listed in table 5.4—as they apply to acquiring and monitoring data necessary for answering these evaluation questions

Because we have already examined analyzing data at length in chapters 3 and 4, and because chapter 6 is devoted to reporting data, the following discussion is restricted to the Socratic elements necessary for acquiring and monitoring data.

What?

The *what* questions you need to answer are, *What types of data are necessary? What specific items need to be measured?* and *What questions must we ask outside vendors in order to secure the data we need?*

Table 5.4   A Data Management Planning Framework

Phase	**Socratic elements**				
	What	**Where**	**Who**	**How**	**When**
Data collection and monitoring	• What type of data will be collected? • What must be measured? • What questions must we ask outside vendors to secure the data we need?	• In-house or out of house? • If out of house, what vendor should be used? • If in-house where is data best collected? • What types of health management databases exist on-site?	• Who will collect the data? • Who will be included in the evaluation: all participants or a random sample of participants?	• How will the data be collected: survey, telephone, interview, personal interview, observation, existing database? • In what format should it be recorded? • Must we establish a baseline in order to evaluate?	• When will the data be collected? • Is an experimental (or non- or quasi-) design involved? • If so, what does it dictate about times of data collection?
Data analysis	• What data collected will be analyzed? • What equipment and materials are needed?	• Where will the data be analyzed?	• Who will analyze the data: one person or a team? • Who will serve as an independent analyst, if needed?	• How will the data be analyzed?	• When will the data be analyzed?
Data reporting	• What analyzed data will be reported? • What type of format will be used to report the data?	• Where will the data be distributed?	• Who will receive the report? • Who is responsible for preparing the report?	• How will results be distributed?	• When will the data be distributed?

What Types of Data Are Necessary?

To begin to decide what data you need, look at the questions you have developed from your goals and objectives, then review chapters 3 and 4 to help you decide what data gathering instruments or analysis tools you will need to answer them. For example, if you want to answer the question, *How many employees have two or more risks for cancer?* you must identify an instrument such as a health risk appraisal or an activity such as medical screenings that will provide this information (see table 5.3). Or, if you want to answer the question, *Is the new health and productivity management campaign meeting employees' health needs and organizational cost-containment goals?* you would need to obtain employee health data that apply to the specific employee health goals that have been established and that measure cost-containment outcomes with various financial accounting tools.

To zero in more precisely on the type of data you would need to gather with the HRA, with the medical screening, from the accounting department, or with employee questionnaires, ask yourself about each goal you are concerned with: *Does this evaluation goal require qualitative or quantitative data? Do I need descriptive or inferential data?*

Qualitative or Quantitative?

A quantitative evaluation produces hard data, such as nominal scores, rankings, frequencies, or classifications. Examples of quantitative data would be the number of participants in a stress management program, the percentage of frequent exercisers, and the baseline number of low back injuries. Programs with variables that can be measured to compare one or more groups against each other or against the general population produce hard data. Financial evaluations use hard data exclusively. Collecting quantitative data will be needed to answer questions such as the following:

- Are men or women more likely to exhibit multiple risk factors for cardiovascular disease?

- What percentage of men versus women exercise at least four days per week?

- Is the new health and productivity management campaign meeting employees' health needs and organizational cost-containment goals?

In contrast, a qualitative evaluation produces soft data, often obtained from interviews, case studies, focus groups, or observations. Qualitative evaluation is suited for programs focused on individual performance or in settings where other descriptive information from participants is needed—for example, stress management. In essence, qualitative data will be needed to answer such questions as

- What is the level of perceived vulnerability in women for developing breast cancer?

- How do men rank their personal heart attack risk compared to their clinical risk?

- What are the most common barriers reported by men versus women for not exercising?

Finally, program evaluators often find advantages to combining quantitative and qualitative methods. For example, combining blood pressure readings of frequent exercisers with interviews of a few participants can strengthen the evaluation. A combined approach is suited for programs that have outcome variables that may be valued differently by various stakeholders. For instance, employees may be more interested in the level of customer service provided by staff members; staff members may be more interested in participation and risk-reduction impacts; and management may be more concerned about health and productivity management outcomes. Specific examples include

- How many employees are completely satisfied with their switch from the traditional fee-for-service indemnity health insurance plan to the new managed care plan?

- What percentage of 20- to 40-year-old female employees participating in the *Preparing for Motherhood* program expressed a higher degree of confidence in their mothering capabilities at the midpoint of the program?

- How many newly diagnosed hypertensive employees have expressed a strong interest in participating in an on-site hypertension control program?

- Is the new health and productivity management campaign meeting employee health needs and organizational cost-containment goals?

Descriptive or Inferential?

Descriptive data supply information about one variable without reference to other variables. For some types of evaluation, descriptive data are appropriate. Here are examples of questions requiring descriptive statistical analyses:

- What is the average age of employees with the highest number of back injury claims?
- What are the three most common occupations represented by EAP users?
- What are the five fastest-growing MDC costs in the past three years?

In contrast, inferential data analysis uses statistical tests to draw tentative conclusions about relationships among variables—for example, how the direction of one variable may influence another. Here are examples of inferential statistical analyses:

- Since health care costs increase at a specific rate when a group's health risk status increases, do health care costs drop proportionately with improved health risk status?
- If repetitive wrist movements are reduced 10%, will the incidence of carpal tunnel syndrome cases drop at a similar rate?

Organizations typically use descriptive data analysis in their initial evaluation projects and incorporate inferential data analysis as the scope of their evaluation broadens. For example, an organization's initial program evaluation may focus primarily on descriptive data such as participants' ages, occupation, and participation levels. Eventually, inferential analyses are performed, such as the relationships between participation and health care costs or between participation and absenteeism.

Be sure that you are familiar with the sources of data that are available to you, such as medical claims, workers' compensation and employee health records, and environmental assessments. Table 5.5 lists types of data and departments where they are typically found in many organizations.

What Items Must Be Measured?

Now that you have an idea of the types of data required to answer your evaluation questions, you need to decide what specific data need to be gathered through already existing records or through measurement of data generated in the future. Again, the questions developed from your general goals are the key.

Table 5.5   Probable Sources of Data Types

Data type	Probable sources					
	Benefits	Human resources	Risk management	Medical	Workers' compensation	Safety
Medical claims (quantitative)	x	x	x			
Workers' compensation (quantitative)	x	x	x	x	x	x
Employee health (quantitative)			x	x	x	
Safety (quantitative)			x	x	x	x
Culture audit (quantitative, qualitative, inferential, descriptive)		x				
Environmental assessment (quantitative, qualitative, inferential, descriptive)				x	x	x

Being aware of the types of data, as discussed previously, serves as a check as you look at what items you've decided to measure. That is, once you look at the items to measure, you check to see if that matches your choice of qualitative/quantitative, descriptive/inferential. If it doesn't match, you need to reevaluate your decision on what to measure.

What Questions Should You Ask Data Sources?

Whether you are collecting data from other departments within your organization or from outside vendors, you must be very specific in your requests. Otherwise, you may end up with statistics that are useless. Again, you must analyze your evaluation goals and target your requests accordingly.

For example, suppose your organization's back injury prevention program is designed to reduce the number of low back injuries among warehouse workers, which have been steadily rising over the past year. All back injury data are currently recorded in the organization's employee benefits department. If you are interested in assessing changes in the cost of low back injuries at your worksite, do not ask the employee benefits officer for *data on the prevalence and cost of back injuries at this worksite*. Rather, ask yourself first, *What is my evaluation goal?* and frame your questions accordingly. Let's assume that your goal is to reduce the prevalence and cost of low back injuries among warehouse workers and that your objections are to (1) provide on-the-job back stretching sessions for all warehouse workers, (2) motivate at least 75% of warehouse workers to increase their back strength and flexibility at least 10% at the end of one month, and (3) generate at least a 20% gain in back strength and flexibility in at least 50% of the workers at the end of six months. Pertinant data includes:

- Data on only employees rather than both employees and dependents
- The total number of low back injuries
- Data that separates statistics on jobs by type of department (e.g., physically demanding versus desk jobs)
- Information from the musculoskeletal MDC, including only the ICDs within it that could correspond to types of low back injury, such as muscle strain or disk disorder
- The age distribution of injured employees—that is, 20-30, 31-40, 41-50, 51 and older
- The activity leading to injury—for example, lifting, reaching, pulling, or pushing
- The types of injuries resulting in recordable time off work
- The most expensive types of back injuries
- The total low back expenses incurred by the organization

If you look at table 5.6, which lists the ICDs within the musculoskeletal MDC, you can see that the irrelevant ICDs have been crossed out. You will have to make similar distinctions within MDCs for many of your evaluations.

Or, say you are requesting claims data reports from outside sources to help you assess whether emergency department visits are a significant factor in rising medical expenses for your organization. When faced with this kind of need, organizations often ask only basic assessment questions, such as the following:

- What are the most common types of claims?
- What are the most expensive types of claims?
- What is the average length of stay for the most common (inpatient) conditions?
- How did this year's overall cost compare with last year's cost?

Table 5.6 A Sample Listing of Musculoskeletal Conditions by ICD

ICD #	Name	Claims (#)	Charges
715.0	Osteoarthritis	15	$4,890
717.9	Int. derange., knee	2	$3,300
719.45	Joint pain, pelvis	3	$1,900
722.1	Lumbar disc disp.	4	$4,900
722.73	Disc disorder	3	$4,500
723.1	Cervicalgia	2	$2,290
724.2	Lumbago	8	$3,200
724.4	Lumbosacral neur.	1	$3,890
724.5	Backache	10	$5,890
726.33	Olecrannon bursitis	3	$3,900
726.64	Patellar tendonitis	2	$3,100
729.5	Pain in limb	3	$1,500
742.59	Spinal cord anomal.	1	$5,900

But the answers to these questions will not enable evaluators to solve the problem of whether emergency room visits are causing your company's rising medical costs. Asking the following problem-focused questions will help evaluators identify the specific cost sources they are concerned about:

- What are the most common claims by major diagnostic category (MDC) and international classification of disease (ICD)?
- How many emergency department claims have been filed in the past three years?
- How does the total number of annual emergency department (ED) claims rank in comparison with other claims?
- What is the most common type of ailment prompting ED usage among employees? Among dependents?
- What percentage of ED claims are filed annually by employees versus dependents?
- What is the average number of ED claims filed annually per employee? Per dependent?
- How does the ED utilization rate compare with local, regional, and national norms?
- What percentage of ED conditions are felt to be linked primarily to lifestyle? Environmental factors? Job-related factors?
- If current ED utilization trends continue, what will the ED rate be in the next three years?

If you are requesting data from either an inside or an outside source, you will then make your job easier if you analyze your data needs in light of your evaluation goals and objectives. You will need to ask questions that will elicit the details you want while excluding data that are unnecessary.

Who?

There are two main questions you must address in the Socratic element *who?* They are, *Who will collect the data?* and *On whom do we need to collect data?*

Who Will Collect the Data?

It is very rare that you will be working entirely alone in planning and implementing WHP evaluation. Even if you are the only WHP employee in your company, or if you are a single consultant doing an evaluation for an organization, you will need to enlist the help of others to collect data in all but the smallest evaluation efforts. After you have identified the data you need, go through your list and write down who you'll need to recruit to help you get each class of information.

For example, basic front-end health screenings—ranging from body-fat analysis to flexibility—require persons who have been formally trained to conduct these procedures. More comprehensive screenings that include exercise stress tests require certified exercise test technologists, exercise physiologists, and other qualified clinicians. People skilled in spreadsheet operations are needed to prepare the files and operate the programs commonly used for data storage, tracking, and analysis.

On Whom Should You Collect Data?

If you are doing a study that involves an experimental, quasi-experimental, or nonexperimental design, that design will tell you the people whose statistics (e.g., blood pressure, participation, heart rate, cholesterol levels) need to be recorded.

Other questions involving data subjects are answered in the process of coming up with targeted questions for data sources, which is discussed in *What Questions Should You Ask Data Sources?*

Where?

Once you have listed all the data you need for whatever evaluations you are planning, you should think about the source for each category of data. Questions to ask yourself are, *Is this data already recorded somewhere (e.g., on medical claims forms)? Do we need to gather it by applying designs to in-house WHP interventions or by creating procedures for keeping appropriate records on segments of company personnel? If it does exist, where is it, and whom do we need to contact to get it? Is the best source in-house or out of house?* Once you reach this level of planning, you may even realize that it is not practical to obtain some of the data you thought you needed. If this is the case, you will need to revise your goals accordingly.

Most midsized and large organizations have in-house systems in place to acquire, record, and monitor health management data such as absenteeism, accidents, program participation, and turnover. In contrast, they usually rely on outside firms (managed care organizations, insurers, and claims administrators) to provide them with medical care, case management, and workers' compensation data. If you need to acquire and monitor employees' attitudes, productivity, and risk factor status changes as regularly as other health management data (which is not often done), it is usually most practical to develop in-house procedures for doing so. In any case, it is vital to be sure that any in-house source from which you need data is aware of what you need and has established suitable procedures for acquiring, recording, and monitoring it. One of the best ways to assure that this happens is for you to develop forms for them to fill out that request the exact information you need. Figure 5.3 illustrates the top section of one such form. If you give your in-house sources a complete set of forms that will provide you with all the data you need if they are correctly filled out, it is more likely that you will get exactly what you need. Figure 5.4 provides a sample form that can be useful for listing all the forms you create for in-house data gathering. For organizational purposes, be sure that each form you create has a clear title and a unique number.

If data would be best obtained from an outside firm, you need to ask about credentials, quality assurance, experience, cost, time lines, credibility of data sources, and references. Review the discussion on pages 57-60 regarding how to choose an outside vendor. Outside sources generally have their own standardized forms on which they record the data you request. In that case, you will need to transfer the numbers from their generic forms onto forms you have created to organize the data in such a way that it answers your very specific questions. These would be similar to the example provided in figure 5.3.

How?

The *how* questions you must deal with are as follows: *How will the data be collected? In what format should it be recorded? Must you establish a baseline in order to evaluate?*

In What Format Should Data Be Recorded?

Data formats can vary considerably from source to source. Some data have to be plugged into a standardized framework because of regulatory mandates such as state or federal occupational safety policies. Thus, on-the-job accidents are recorded on standardized formats that are approved and monitored by officials at both levels. Some instruments such as health risk appraisals (HRAs) contain data with similar formats that may differ in one or more features. For instance, most HRA formats contain data on a person's demographic background and lifestyle behaviors, yet, they often vary in content, length, and methodologies used to estimate personal risk. Health management data formats used to record and track absenteeism, employee assistance services, case management, productivity, turnover, and other performance measures are generally developed by in-house staff who prefer to use tools and techniques that can be customized to fit their own organization. When creating customizing data formats, decision makers should consider the following factors:

- Types of outcomes data of greatest value to the organization (e.g., absenteeism, risk factor status, productivity)

Major diagnostic category	Number of claims	Total charges	Average charge per claim	Total charges paid
Accidents/injuries and poisoning	35	$ 3,500	$ 100	$ 2,800
Circulatory	100	100,500	1,005	90,000
Digestive	58	35,000	604	30,000
End/Nut/Metab	37	27,500	743	21,400
Female reproductive	23	10,900	473	9,100
Musculoskeletal	150	90,000	600	79,100
Pregnancy	24	53,200	2,216	46,000
Respiratory	30	20,000	666	17,500

Figure 5.3 An abbreviated version of a sample medical care claims and cost data collection form.

Type of data	Acquisition		Monitoring	
	In-house	Out of house	In-house	Out of house
Absenteeism				
Accidents/injuries				
Attitude/morale (job satisfaction)				
Case management				
Medical care claims and charges				
Participation				
Productivity				
Risk factor status				
Turnover				
Workers' compensation				

Figure 5.4 A sample planning worksheet to record forms needed to acquire and monitor health management data.

- Level of data existing on current formats
- Level of data needed on new formats
- How often specific types of data are needed
- Who will use specific types of data

Third-party vendors (insurers and claims administrators, in particular) often have computerized resources to tabulate, code, and analyze health management data for their employer clients. For example, many health insurers and claims administrators prepare medical claims data in spreadsheet and graphic-oriented formats that enable their clients to perform specific analyses.

Sometimes it is difficult to know what formats to request from a third-party vendor. In such cases, ask the vendor what types of formats currently exist and, if possible, to show you samples you can compare to determine which format most closely resembles your needs. You can often adapt formats that are not exactly what you need. For example, table 5.7 is the first few rows of a claims data spreadsheet provided to an organization by its claims administrator. The full sheet includes the 50 most expensive types of claims. Notice the rows of data have been summed into their respective totals. While this is useful information, suppose that you are also interested in knowing the average amount paid per claim to identify, say, the ten claims that have the highest average cost. Since this is a spreadsheet application, you could easily add a new column, I (average cost per claim), and calculate those averages by dividing column H (paid) by column G (total number of claims).

Must We Establish a Baseline in Order to Evaluate?

What if you have been asked to do a break-even analysis of a program designed to reduce the prevalence of risk factors for cancer but have been given no information about which risk factors were most prevalent in the workforce before the current program was put into place? In this case, you must, of course, establish a baseline before you can proceed with the evaluation. For some evaluations, such as this one, you can ask the occupational health nurse to review employees' medical histories and health risk appraisal data to identify the most common risk factors to use as a baseline.

For other evaluations, such as gauging the level of participant satisfaction in specific programs, it will be necessary to do a pilot assessment or a pilot test. These are instruments for gathering pre-intervention information from a representative sample of a target population. This information is absolutely necessary for certain assessments. For instance, suppose you have been asked to evaluate participant opinions of fitness center staff. To do this, you will need a baseline measure of satisfaction levels, but no such measurements have been made. In this case, you could develop a one-page survey and randomly administer it to a portion of program participants. The data can then be tabulated, formatted, and used as a baseline level of participant satisfaction.

Table 5.7 Section of Sample Claims Data Report

	A	B	C	D	E	F	G	H
				Employee			Total	
			Male		Female			
	Code	Description	Claims (#)	Paid ($)	Claims (#)	Paid ($)	Claims (#)	Paid ($)
1	1629-1629	Mal neo bronch/lung	182	17,939	986	141,955	1,168	159,894
2	78650-78650	Chest pain nos	119	24,875	707	119,211	826	144,086
3	650-650	Normal delivery	0	0	203	134,534	203	134,534
4	325-325	Phlebitis intrcran s	0	0	24	131,209	24	131,209
5	57410-57410	Cholelith w cholecys	19	9,283	104	118,015	123	127,298
6	1749-1749	Malign neopl breast	0	0	498	113,347	498	113,347
7	7100-7100	Syst lupus erythemat	0	0	694	107,108	694	107,108
8	5751-5751	Cholecystitis nec	7	11,109	94	91,152	101	102,261
9	71596-71596	Osteoarthros nos-l/l	8	305	155	92,981	163	93,286
10	41401-41401	Rnry athrscl natve v	32	17,430	41	71,043	73	88,473

What to Do If Data Arrive in Wrong Format

If you have been careful about your selection of outside vendors, and if you have asked them and your internal sources the right questions, you will usually receive reports that contain the data you need in a format you can use. However, if you are coming into a situation that you have not been able to control from the outset (if, for example, you are a consultant, or have been hired by a company in the middle of the fiscal/evaluation year), it is likely that

- you will receive data reports that are not ideal in either content or format or
- you will be given reports and will be expected to perform whatever analyses you can based on what you've got.

In either case, your first step must be to review the data to determine if a basic assessment or a comprehensive problem-focused analysis can be done with what you have received. For instance, if the data on an in-house program include participants' gender, age, and participation levels for six consecutive months, you could perform more analyses than if the data were limited to a single month. You will often find that in order to do any analysis at all, the data must be cleaned, reduced, coded, and transposed into a usable format. Data from surveys and observation sheets, for example, may have to be coded and entered into a database to be analyzed. Sometimes even these measures will not yield the data you need. In these cases, you should try to get what you need rather than limiting yourself to what you have been given.

> **Computer Tip**
>
> Various software programs contain scheduling framework and forms to enhance program planning and evaluation efforts. Before purchasing any software package, take time to develop your evaluation goals, identify the scope and specificity of existing evaluation data, determine what time frame intervals you plan to use, and what features the new software should provide compared to your existing package. Finally, request samples from several manufacturers to see how their software works and whether it will meet your needs.

When?

The final issue you must deal with planning data management is scheduling. Ideally, you should establish a master schedule. Specifically, you must know when your deadlines for various evaluations are and schedule your data acquisition, tabulation, analysis, and presentations accordingly. Be sure to schedule enough time for troubleshooting, such as having to deal with data requests unsatisfactorily met or dependable personnel deciding to leave the company.

Many data acquisition scheduling points will be determined for you by the scheduling work that has been done on planning WHP programs, such as interventions that have an experimental, quasi-experimental, or non-experimental design assigned to them, or evaluations that already have monthly, quarterly, or semiannual data collections specified. Be sure that you have provided those who will be recording the data with tabulation sheets that include the dates or date ranges for them to be filled in. Depending on the requirements of the evaluation, such sheets need not be complex (see figure 5.5).

	Claims (utilization)		Charges	
MDC	Employees (#)	Dependents (#)	Employees ($)	Dependents ($)
Circulatory Hypertension Angina pectoris Ischemia				
Musculo-skeletal Lumbago Arthritis Bursitis				
Respiratory Bronchitis Influenza Asthma				

Figure 5.5 A sample tabulation sheet.

REVIEW QUESTIONS: DESIGN SELECTION AND DATA MANAGEMENT

1. Give several examples of how the purpose of and resources for an evaluation will affect design selection in the event a design is required.
2. What are three essential tasks involving data that must be done if evaluation is to be successful?
3. What three things should be kept in mind as you plan evaluation data management?
4. Discuss the five Socratic questions as they relate to WHP evaluation data management.
5. What factors should be considered before purchasing any scheduling software?

CHAPTER REVIEW

Summary

In planning an evaluation, it is important to consider who the stakeholders are and what immediate or subsequent investments they have in the program. By doing so, you can establish clearly delineated goals relevant to their individual and collective needs and interests. Some stakeholders have a greater interest in health-related goals

(continued)

while other stakeholders are more interested in hard-line financial goals. In using both types of goals within an evaluation, it is vital to establish tangible objectives to specify what actions are required to achieve each goal. Resources—ranging from personnel to equipment—must be secured to put these objectives into motion. Finally, the Socratic approach (who, what, where, when, and how) can be used to generate objective findings to enhance future programming decisions. The *Planning Form for Goal Assessment* (page 137) can help you visualize the steps you need to take and the resources you will need to plan your evaluation of program goals using the information presented in this chapter. If you would find it helpful, you may copy the form and use it in your evaluation planning.

What Would You Do?

You and your colleagues are planning an evaluation of a new fatigue-prevention program that will begin soon in your trucking company. Several colleagues propose an evaluation plan framework consisting of three major steps. First, they propose that on-site and off-site evaluation resources be identified. Second, they propose that an evaluation design be determined that will incorporate participants and nonparticipants. Finally, they propose that outcome measures (dependent variables) be developed to determine any impact of the program. They believe that using these three steps will streamline the evaluation process and save personnel, equipment, and financial resources. You note that this condensed approach is missing several key steps that standard evaluation frameworks include. You also diplomatically point out that the three proposed steps are not properly sequenced and will thus compromise the quality and credibility of any evaluation. They ask you to suggest a more comprehensive approach that is still economical. What would you propose?

6

Preparing and Presenting Evaluation Results

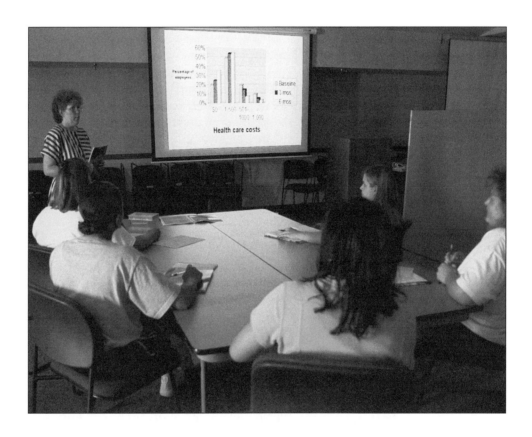

After reading this chapter and answering the questions at the end, you should be able to do the following:

- Identify various issues to address while interpreting cost-related data.

- List several types of stakeholders.

- Describe the value of providing regular progress reports to specific stakeholders.

- List several factors to consider when formatting an evaluation report.

- Describe preliminary considerations in preparing a clear presentation of data.

- List several steps to follow in making a successful presentation.

- Describe how to enhance the utilization of evaluation results.

In the last chapter, we listed the three data-related tasks of evaluation as

- acquiring and monitoring data,
- analyzing data (which is discussed in chapters 3 and 4), and
- reporting data.

Acquiring and monitoring data are extensively discussed in chapter 5. This chapter deals with issues of analyzing data not covered in chapters 3 and 4, and it also discusses how to present data in evaluation reports. We begin with interpreting results, moving then to identifying and targeting stakeholders, and finally presenting and applying evaluation results.

Interpreting Results

Once the results of analyses are available, evaluators must interpret them to answer each evaluation question. Interpretation is more than simply reviewing the results to determine if the intervention made an impact on the dependent variable. It is also exploring the significance of any impact and identifying possible factors that directly and indirectly could have influenced the impact or lack thereof. In this section we consider program significance versus statistical significance and problems to be aware of when interpreting cost data on populations you are investigating and when looking for trends.

Program Significance Versus Statistical Significance

The interpretation of evaluation results should distinguish between program significance (practical significance) and statistical significance. **Program significance** is the usefulness of an observation whereas **statistical significance** is a probability statement about its accuracy. Statistical significance is similar to reliability (consistency) in that they are both measures of precision.

It is important to distinguish between statistical significance and program significance. It is possible for an evaluation to show statistically significant positive results yet for the program significance of those same statistics (particularly when combined with economic analysis) to be negative. For example, suppose that a large number of workers have recently completed a six-month intervention designed to (a) build observance of proper lifting techniques and (b) reduce low back injury costs. Back injury costs were tracked at three intervals: at two months, at four months, and at six months. Low back injury costs were reduced by 1% at two months, 3% at four months, and 4% at six months. Supervisory observations at each of the three intervals revealed that improvements in lifting techniques among program participants improved at similar rates. However, when cost effectiveness and break-even analysis were applied to the program, the evaluators discovered that the intervention cost to produce these minor improvements was far more than the economic benefits and that projections did not suggest any improvement in the economic picture. Once econometric analyses were done, program planners concluded that the program should be drastically redesigned or dropped—despite the statistically significant positive impact of the program on both lower back injury costs and workers' practice of proper lifting techniques.

Cost Data on Populations

Interpreting and reporting cost data on populations presents unique challenges. To analyze, interpret, and report cost data accurately on human subjects, evaluators should do the following:

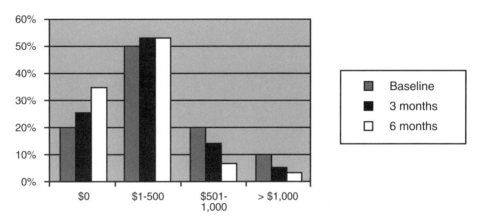

Figure 6.1   Health care cost distribution by percentage of employees at baseline, three months, and six months.

- **Report the distribution of costs.** For example, how significant is the change in the slope (skewness) from baseline to outcome? Figure 6.1 illustrates health care costs at specific intervals that show more wide-scale distribution at the baseline compared with six months. This pattern reveals that a higher percentage of high-cost users at baseline moved to a lower cost trend over the designated time frame.

- **Separate cost information by potentially significant variables.** Report any differences among groups regarding gender, age, ethnicity, body composition, health-related habits, or any other variables that you suspect may be significant. If such data are not available, question whether these variables may have influenced the results.

- **If possible, compare your data against a reliable baseline.** If possible, use several years of data to establish your baseline. Note the degree of variation within the baseline data over time between different ethnic or occupational groups, or according to whatever other factors are appropriate for the study you are doing.

- **Recognize that total cost also hides individual differences.** Total costs do not necessarily indicate differences among individuals as any difference could be due to a few expensive individuals or a small cost difference among many group members. Ways to deal with this fact include the following:

  - **Interpret means (averages) with caution.** It is tempting to interpret a difference in means as a difference between two separate groups. This assumption implies that all members of the more costly group cost more than members of the less costly group. The presence of extreme cases (outliers) will invalidate this assumption.

  - **Compare medians.** Recall that the median is a midpoint that 50% of the scores are above and 50% of the scores are below. Compare the difference among group-to-group medians to see if they are similar to or different from any differences in means. In most cases, differences in medians among groups are more accurate indicators of real differences among group members. Medians are less likely to be influenced by extremely high or low scores than means as shown in table 6.1.

  - **Identify and note the percentage of employees incurring low or no costs.** Any difference in the percentage of employees in experimental groups having no medical claim costs will influence the mean. For example, note in figure 6.1 that 35% of the employees had no costs at six months compared to 20% at the baseline. Such a significant increase in no-cost employees will normally result in a lower median and a lower mean as long as the remaining employees do not substantially increase their expenses.

Table 6.1 Median Versus Mean

Group A		Group B
$1,000		$5,000
$ 800		$2,500
$ 750		$1,000
$ 650		$ 750
$ 650		$ 600
$ 562	Median	$ 550
$ 475		$ 500
$ 275		$ 475
$ 275		$ 275
$ 100		$ 100
$ 75		$ 75
$5,612	Total	$11,275
$ 510	Mean	$ 1,006

- **Interpret statistical significance cautiously.** Different types of statistical tests are designed to deal with different types of data; thus, there are certain tests designed to deal with skewness and certain tests that aren't. If your data does feature skewness, be sure you use an appropriate test. For example, statistical analysis tests such as analysis of variance (ANOVA), analysis of co-variance (CO-ANOVA), chi-square analysis, multivariate analysis, and multiple regression analysis can measure skewness and related variable measures. Also, note the strength of significance levels and the likelihood that outside (extraneous) variables could have contributed to the significant outcome.

The preceding examples should make it very clear that interpreting cost data is extremely complex. Therefore, beginners (or even nonbeginners faced with an unusually complex situation) should consult with statisticians if they have the resources to do so.

Identifying Trends

When the value of a variable changes in a consistent direction over time (upward or downward), a trend may be evolving. It is important to identify and report trends in an evaluation. They are useful in doing long-term forecasting to determine future participation, compliance rates, risk factor prevalence, cost-savings, and other prospective outcomes (see chapter 4).

Computer Tip

When dealing with rows and columns of data, use a spreadsheet program to perform quick calculations that may or may not require a specific formula. For example, consecutive rows or columns of data can be automatically summed by first highlighting the selected rows or columns and then tapping on the sum sign ( ) with y our cursor. Of course, additional calculations such as subtraction, division, multiplication, averages, and standard deviations, to mention a few, can be performed by simply inserting the appropriate formula that is available in the Help, Index, or Search sections on your desktop menu.

A Stitch in Time

In its initial two years of operation, an East Coast hospital-based health promotion program included various nonfinancial incentives to motivate employee participation. During the third year of the program, staff members noted a steady month-to-month decline in participation from a 5% drop in May to nearly a 30% drop by August. Some staff members speculated that warmer weather and summer vacations were primarily responsible for the downturn. Other staff noted, however, that similar declines had not occurred in the two previous years. Rather than waiting to see if this trend would continue into the fall, the program director immediately

- offered more individually based programs rather than team/group activities,
- developed an on-site walking/jogging trail, and
- provided financial incentives for regular participation, in consultation with the benefits department.

By virtue of acting quickly to stem the short-term drop-off, program staff were able to market an enhanced program, recovering 70% of the original group of participants. In contrast, had the short-term trend continued into the fall, at least 50% of the initial group of participants would have likely quit the program. By promptly recognizing the downward participation trend, the program director was able to act before participation dwindled to a point at which the future of the program could have been jeopardized.

However, what may appear to be a definite trend in one setting may be viewed as nothing more than a temporary change in another. A trend may only be in the eye of the beholder if evaluators do not establish objective criteria to clearly define it. Take a look at figures 6.2 and 6.3, which show variations of a trend. Figure 6.2 shows a consistent weekly improvement in low back flexibility. When changes occur in the same direction without interruption through an extended period of time, a continuous trend is evident. In contrast, figure 6.3 exhibits **variable trending** patterns because the degree of change from interval to interval is not consistent.

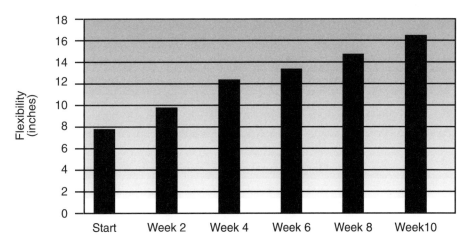

Figure 6.2   A sample continuous trend from start to week 10 indicating average low back flexibility.

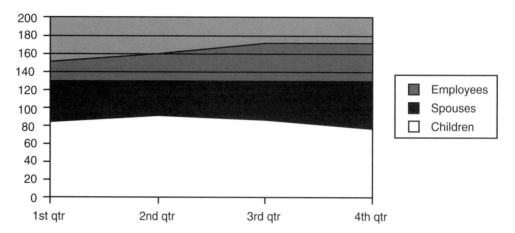

Figure 6.3 An illustration of variable trending showing the total number of quarterly health care visits by group.

As shown in figure 6.3, trends can differ in their onset, direction (**skewness**), duration, or degree of linear change (**kurtosis**). These factors should be considered when evaluating both employee health and organizational health variables. For example, what may be perceived initially as a possible trend might be instead a seasonal fluctuation or a naturally occurring event. To decide which of these is the case, it may be necessary to compare several shorter intervals over a longer time frame to determine if a trend is due to seasonal factors or other natural events that require more investigation. The length of the longer time frame will depend on what cyclical events could affect any possible confounding factors.

Trends develop at different rates for different types of variables. Employee health variables such as blood pressure, cholesterol, and exercise levels can be improved in a few weeks with appropriate interventions whereas organizational health outcomes such as absenteeism, health care cost management, and productivity are usually held to a higher standard. Organizational health outcomes tend to fluctuate more than employee health status indicators and are often influenced significantly by external forces such as the national or regional economy. Therefore, many evaluators will not consider changes in an organizational health outcome as a real trend unless the change is consistently longer or sharper than an employee health trend.

Certain factors are often associated with certain time frames that must be achieved by a direction of development before it can be considered a trend. Consider the following examples:

- **Short-term** (1-6 months)
    - Accidents/injuries
    - Attitude/morale
    - Health care utilization (emergency department usage)
    - Risk factor status (blood pressure, blood glucose, exercise)
- **Intermediate** (7-12 months)
    - Absenteeism
    - Case management
    - Health care utilization (overall)
    - Risk factor status (serum cholesterol, drug use)
    - Productivity
    - Workers' comp claims

- **Long-term** (> 12 months)
  - Health care charges
  - Workers' comp charges

Identifying Stakeholders and Their Needs

As is the case in so many aspects of evaluation, the process of reporting results must begin with your stakeholders. No matter how good your WHP program may be, if your reports are not targeted at the needs and interests of those who make the decisions in that program (from intervention participants to those who set budgets), your WHP evaluation efforts will most likely be ineffective, which will eventually result in the downgrading and deterioration of the health promotion program itself.

If you have designed your WHP programs and their evaluations properly, you will have begun by identifying your stakeholders. These same stakeholders must all be addressed directly in your evaluations, and each interested party (whether individual or group) should receive reports that are specific to its needs. Figure 6.4 illustrates an excellent flowchart developed by the Association for Worksite Health Promotion to show how communication should work in WHP evaluation.

It is vital that in your reports to each group, you address the concerns listed below it. If you do not, you are likely to end up with management who do not want to fund the program, a planning committee that is confused about what to do, and employees who have no interest in participating. On the other hand, if you discuss each of these concerns appropriately, you will have management who understand and support the program, a planning committee that works effectively, and employees who participate with enthusiasm and reap all the health and wellness benefits you want them to have. Let's look at each of these groups in more detail.

Who Should Know What?

WHP staff at a southwestern oil and gas exploration company attribute much of their success to targeting their evaluation reports to key stakeholder groups. For example, participation and risk-reduction data are tracked on a monthly basis and shared with management at quarterly intervals; program participants receive monthly progress reports on their individual goals; the program planning committee receives quarterly reports throughout the year on programming elements such as number of programs offered, participation, compliance rates, penetration impact, and user satisfaction data. Finally, cash flow status data is prepared monthly on spreadsheet formats and submitted to the human resources director and chief financial officer at quarterly intervals. This multilevel reporting system consistently provides key stakeholders with timely information that is critical for the ongoing success of the company's WHP program.

(continued)

(continued)

In contrast, misguided reporting efforts can seriously jeopardize a WHP program. The program director at a northeastern telecommunications company made this near-fatal mistake and almost caused the demise of the company's year-old program. Failing to understand the varied interests of all stakeholders, he designed program evaluations exclusively around employee health status indicators. Consequently, the evaluation results were of little, if any, value to management, employee committee members, or staff members. Fortunately, a senior manager who was interested in the success of WHP in the company diplomatically informed the program director of this reporting oversight. In response, the program director quickly reassessed stakeholders' interests, designed a broadened evaluation framework with appropriate instruments, and prepared several evaluation reports tailored to the specific interests of each stakeholder group. WHP at his company is no longer at risk.

Management

Most senior managers do not care about day-to-day work plans. They want to know about the bottom line. Is the program financially justifiable? Are the workers healthier and more productive with the program than without it? Is it adding to the company's profitability—if not, does it provide other tangible benefits that make it worth retaining or expanding, or is it moving in the direction of increasing profitability?

Managers are likely to be interested in reports containing information regarding progress toward general goals related to long-range plans. To ensure that you are addressing all possible interests, go back and review any brainstorming sessions you had with management when you were planning the program and its evaluation.

Of particular importance are goals that are not likely to be attained in the designated time frame. As with budget problems, the reporting manager should be prepared to provide a brief explanation of perceived barriers and how they can be addressed in the future. Not only is negative information not to be ignored, it should, in a sense, be emphasized because it shows where things need improvement. For example, you should point out programs that are not currently profitable, then either discuss the measures that are being taken to make them so or show clearly when the current trend is likely to result in profitability and why you think that trend will continue. You should preempt negativity by identifying current and possible problems, and suggest solutions.

When possible, gather background information on the managers who will be receiving the evaluation report: What is their educational background? Do they participate in the program? Do they prefer more information on the process of evaluation or simply the bottom-line outcomes? Do they prefer narrative or graphic-oriented reports? Are certain managers more likely to receive and closely review the report, such as human resources, benefits, safety, and medical personnel? If so, does the report include results of particular value to each of these individuals? For example, if a particular manager spearheaded financial support for the expansion of a new health promotion facility, the level of participation in the facility may be very important politically to that executive. Finally, reports submitted to management should invite managers to participate in programs. If you have done your homework, you'll know which managers are likely to be interested in which interventions. The more you can get them involved, of course, the more likely it is that they will understand the value of the programs, and the more support they will give you.

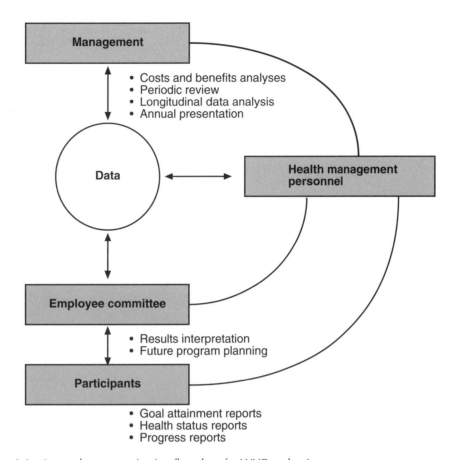

Figure 6.4 A sample communication flowchart for WHP evaluation.
Reprinted, by permission, from Association for Fitness in Business, 1992. *Guidelines for employee health promotion programs* (Champaign, IL: Human Kinetics), 75.

Employee Committee and Program Participants

The committee usually consists of employees who participate in the WHP program. They are most often interested in evaluation data relevant to participants' interests. They generally have opinions and recommendations to share with program decision makers. They often interpret results from HRAs, culture audits, and environmental health check sheets to help determine the direction of future programs.

Directly soliciting regular feedback from participating employees as well as providing consistent reports to them fosters ownership and ongoing commitment. Participants are very interested in their personal health status and performance indicators such as blood pressure, heart disease risk, and overall fitness level.

Reporting Evaluation Results

It is important that you understand not only how to prepare both written and oral reports, but also how to take the political situation into account as you present your reports.

Preparing Written Reports

Many organizations and departments have guidelines for constructing evaluation reports, but in others, any format is acceptable as long as it communicates the information clearly. Formats may include technical reports, journal articles, employee newsletters, news releases, meetings, departmental memos, presentations, press conferences, personal letters, or workshops. Generally, more than one method of communication is used to meet the needs of all stakeholders. For example, following a new worksite health promotion program, staff members may prepare an executive summary for management, an e-mail memo to thank all participating employees, a news release to the local television station, and a technical report to the funding source (if outside funding was obtained).

Progress Reports

Progress reporting completes the loop between planning and the daily flow of work. Progress reports may be formal or informal, ranging from scheduled presentations to informal telephone calls. If they are to be effective, they must be submitted on time to provide immediate feedback so appropriate program modifications can be made. For example, process evaluations in a one-year back injury prevention program may be conducted at two-month intervals to provide staff members with opportunities to scrutinize the intervention and make adjustments, as needed. See the sample condensed monthly report in *Corporate Monthly Report*.

Corporate Monthly Report

During March, we experienced a 4% increase in participation from February (from 1,341 to 1,292). Last year, the increase in participation from February to March was only 2% (from 1,375 to 1,391). The 2% difference is reflective of this year's programming strategy that has marketed and implemented the spring activities as a sequence of events. In the previous year, these same events were clustered together, and March was the peak participation month. Specific progress indicators include the following:

- Daily attendance dropped by 10.5% in the past year.
- Fifty-two percent (52%) or 1,341 employees of the downtown site utilized the program during March.
- Our new Mileage Challenge Club has a total of 238 participants.
- CPR was the most popular program, followed by stress management, weight management, low back pain, and allergies.
- Our first Associate Membership Health Fair was held and well-received by employees. One hundred and twenty (120) reply cards have been received from interested employees.
- Fat Chance Weight Management program was initiated the last week in March with a captain's meeting.
- Seven (7) employees were counseled on weight control and nutrition in March.

Hard-Copy Program Effectiveness Reports

A hard-copy report provides program staff and evaluators with an opportunity to present a detailed overview of significant events that occurred during each phase of the evaluation, as well as the results and conclusions. The typical components of a written report on a program effectiveness evaluation, as well as of econometric reports, are the following:

- **Abstract/executive summary** provides an overview of the intervention and its evaluation, including general results, conclusions, and recommendations. See *Abstract*, below, for a sample abstract.

- **Table of contents** lists sections with their page numbers.

- **Introduction** discusses the purpose of the evaluation, program and participant description, goals and objectives of the intervention, and evaluation questions that were used.

- **Methods/procedures** explains the evaluation design (when one was used), target population (participants, nonparticipants), instruments (surveys, risk appraisals), sampling procedures, databases, data collection procedures, pilot study results (if applicable), methods used to improve validity and reliability, limitations and assumptions of the evaluation process, and procedures for analyzing data.

- **Results/outcomes** describes and explains findings, answers to evaluation questions, comparisons against norms (industry, national), and includes graphic illustrations of findings (charts, tables).

- **Conclusions/recommendations** interprets the results by explaining the level of intervention effectiveness, the recommendations (intervention and staff), and considerations for the future.

- **References** enumerates the sources used (journals, databases).

- **Appendixes** include the data and forms that are too bulky for the main body.

Abstract

Pregnancy-related charges are the largest single component of health-care costs for our organization. Fortunately, many of the risk factors associated with preterm and low birth-weight infants are modifiable. This study examines the impact of an incentive-based worksite prenatal education program on pregnancy-related medical costs and birth weight at HMA Corporation from 1996 to 1999. The 191 program class participants were compared to the 815 nonparticipants. The average medical cost per delivery for participants was $9,245, and the average cost for nonparticipants was $10,936. The rate of participants who had a cesarean section delivery was 16.2% while the rate was 22.2% among nonparticipants. Class participants had fewer low birth-weight and preterm deliveries (3.1%) than nonpartici-pants (4.1%). HMA's prenatal education program has demonstrated that a significant financial incentive is necessary for participation. Workplace prenatal education classes could result in significant savings in health and disability savings for the company.

Preparing a Successful Oral Presentation

Once an evaluation report has been developed, it is often appropriate to present it orally to various stakeholders. Speaking before a group is a learned skill—one that sometimes takes years of training. To make an effective presentation you must know your subject, set and meet high standards, and prepare conscientiously.

Completing the following seven steps will substantially increase your chances of making a powerful oral presentation:

1. **Identify the primary purpose of your presentation.** Is it to inform or instruct? Is it to sell or persuade? Is it to generate awareness? Is it to interpret or clarify? Is it to

make recommendations? Although most evaluation presentations have several objectives, it is important to determine which ones merit the greatest consideration with each audience.

2. **Know your audience.** If you understand what interests and motivates your audience, you can tailor the presentation data, style, and audiovisuals more effectively for them. For instance, what is the average education level of the audience? How familiar are they with the program? Do they participate in the program?

Illustrating a Break-Even Point

The same data can be illustrated in several ways. Here are three different graphs illustrating the same break-even point data. One way is to use a graph featuring different lines to illustrate changes in different items on the same grid, as shown in figure 6.5. A second way is to create a chart that contains two bars at each interval: The bar appearing on the left side at each point signifies the value of one factor while the bar appearing on the right side at the same point signifies the value of another. In the case of this BEA data, the bar representing benefits exceeds the bar representing costs in the third quarter, at which time the break-even point has been achieved, as in figure 6.6. Finally, the same break-even point can also be highlighted using contrasting linear grids whereby the cost-savings grid pattern meets and crosses over the program intervention cost pattern, as figure 6.7 illustrates.

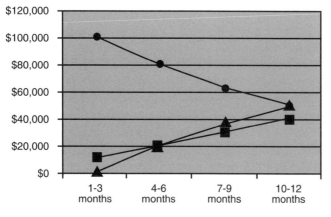
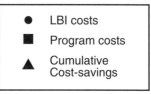

Figure 6.5   Using a line graph.

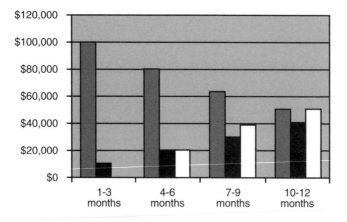
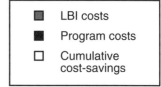

Figure 6.6   Using a bar graph.

(continued)

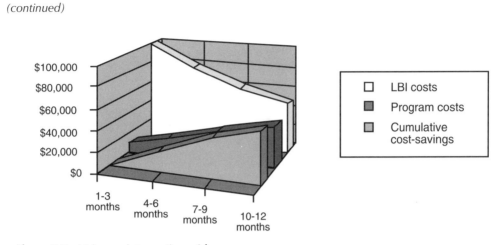

Figure 6.7   Using an intersecting grid.

3. **Decide what to include in the presentation.** What information does the audience need to know? What information is irrelevant to them? Is there something that could be easily misinterpreted or controversial? Consider the six Socratic questions (who, what, where, when, why, and how). Decide which of them are relevant to each topic you have decided to discuss and take the time to answer those questions fully.

4. **Thoroughly study and digest the evaluation data you will be presenting.** Discussing all the data and evaluation results with colleagues can often shed new light on what the real outcomes are and how best to present them.

5. **Organize your material.** Some presenters prefer to organize the presentation by starting with the introduction and proceeding to the end. Other presenters organize their material by starting at the end and working backward to the start. Whatever approach you take, be sure that each section of your presentation is limited to one topic and that it has been preceded by whatever information is necessary for the audience to understand it. Be sure that there is a clear rationale for the order in which you present the topics, whether it be chronological, analytical, or for emotional effect. Be sure that you yourself understand that rationale and how the progression of your presentation supports it. This will enable you to shape your ideas and the evaluation results into a continuous, flowing script.

6. **Decide what audiovisual aids you need and where to use them.** Audiences like visually appealing graphics such as pie charts and bar graphs that illustrate key outcomes. Be sure that you have included all the labels, figures, and caption information necessary to make your graphics clear (see figure 6.8). Commonly used audiovisual equipment includes the overhead transparency projector, carousel slide projector, videocassette player, and LCD projector. It is good to have a backup system in case the primary system fails. For example, if you're using an LCD projector and it malfunctions, have a carousel slide projector or an overhead transparency projector on hand as a backup. You should, of course, be sure that you can operate

Computer Tip

Virtually all of today's software programs have standard features that allow you to automatically convert a table into a graphic illustration. A typical conversion includes these steps:

1. Click on a table framework in the toolbar.

2. Complete the necessary rows and columns with appropriate data.

3. Click on the graph icon in the toolbar, which will present the data in a specific graphic illustration (i.e., bar, lines, pie chart).

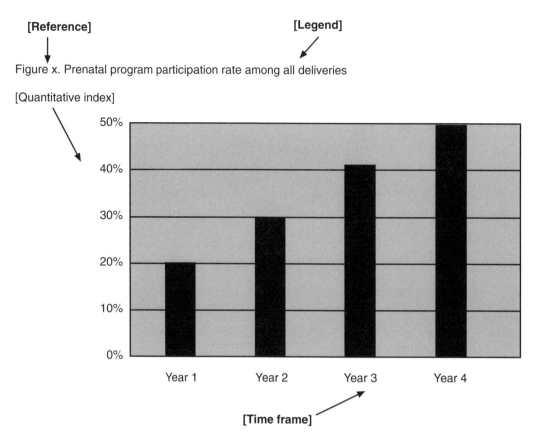

[Reference]

[Legend]

Figure x. Prenatal program participation rate among all deliveries

[Quantitative index]

[Time frame]

Figure 6.8 Example of detailed graphic illustration.

the equipment or that you have an assistant who can do so. Finally, printed handouts distributed to the audience should include key data and graphics.

7. **Practice.** Finally, rehearse your presentation several times to identify and correct potential pitfalls. Do it at least once with the visual aids and audio visual equipment. If possible, find out where the presentation is scheduled and evaluate the physical setup of the area—for instance, size and shape of room, seating arrangement, availability of audiovisual equipment, and lighting. Also, prepare for the prospect of answering questions during or after the presentation.

Taking Politics Into Account

Consider both timing and the decision-making climate in presenting both written and oral evaluation reports. If you are not careful how you present results, you may create distrust among staff members, or you could submit a written report that would never be read by the intended audience. There are, however, several ways you can minimize such possibilities:

- Give key decision makers advance information on the evaluation results, particularly when they are unexpected. If you avoid surprising decision makers in a public forum, you will increase the likelihood that the information will be respected and used at an appropriate time.

- Provide and maintain anonymity and confidentiality of people and organizations at all times. This privacy is particularly vital when dealing with medical claims data, medical records data, and employee assistance program (EAP) data.

- Always do your homework on your audience. Know their interests and identify ways to target your phrasing of evaluation results at what they perceive to be their most important needs. Be sure to provide all information that is pertinent to the group you are addressing in each presentation, whether in oral or written form.

Even negative results can offer valuable information to program staff when viewed in the proper context. Such results usually indicate some shortfall in the conceptualization, planning, marketing, implementation, or evaluation phase of an intervention. Typical causes of negative results include the following:

- Incompetent instructors
- Inadequate incentives
- Lack of participants' ownership of program
- Inefficient operations and administration
- Interventions that lack substance and perceived value
- Inadequate resources—personnel, equipment, facilities
- Inappropriate testing procedures—validity and reliability issues
- Insufficient time for program intervention to affect outcome variable
- Inappropriate evaluation methodologies used
- Incompetent personnel used to analyzed and interpret evaluation data

Though no one likes negative results, evaluations that show program failures or negative trends are among the most valuable assessments you will do. It is not only unethical, but also ineffective to stifle unfavorable results. It is vital to present them in such a way that their value is clear. Always indicate how applying negative results can have positive benefits. Do the results suggest how an ineffective program can be made effective? Do they suggest it should be dropped altogether? Do they show that the WHP program needs to revisit its priorities? Such results are just as important as those that show that things are going well and need to continue in the same direction. Whether results are positive or negative does not affect their usefulness. What is crucial is that they be accurate so that management can revise the design, marketing, or administration of current interventions as necessary, and so that they can plan new ones intelligently. It is up to the evaluation team to present results in such a way that the organization can understand how positive programs can be strengthened and can identify weaknesses of and possible remedies for those programs that are not going as well.

REVIEW QUESTIONS: IDENTIFYING STAKEHOLDERS AND THEIR NEEDS AND REPORTING EVALUATION RESULTS

1. How might stakeholder groups differ in their evaluation needs and interests?
2. What purpose do progress reports serve, and what information should they include?
3. What steps should be taken to make a successful oral presentation?
4. How can an evaluation report be structured to enhance the prospect that the results will be utilized?

Applying Evaluation Results

Far too often, evaluation reports will be submitted to decision makers, but the recommendations will not be implemented. Sometimes, the reasons for failure are beyond the control of evaluators and program staff. For instance, decision makers may not use findings because they are conducting the evaluation only to fulfill requirements of the funding source. Other reasons include that they want to serve their own self-interest and bias or gain recognition for a program. Perhaps they simply believe the costs of implementing the recommendations are prohibitively high. Even decision makers who do plan to use the evaluation results in their health promotion program may find that they are unable to interpret the results or recommendations properly due to their technicality or applicability to a specific individual or department. Following the guidelines below will increase the probability that evaluation results will be used:

- **Follow the principles of effective evaluation planning and execution that have been presented in this text.** If you study this text carefully and incorporate all the principles it teaches into your evaluation planning and implementation, you will provide your employer with accurate information that will prove its own worth over time.

- **Offer specific recommendations based on specific results.** For example, if you have done a comprehensive report summarizing the results of all the WHP evaluations of the previous year, you could pull from that report all the results that suggest what standards would be both effective and achievable for various aspects of the WHP program. *Recommended Standards* is an example of standards that are advocated and the evaluation results that suggested them.

- **Offer recommendations that are within the power of decision makers to implement.** When making recommendations to specific decision makers, be sure they have the power and ability to implement them. A recommendation to expand the company's medical self-care program, which will require more financial resources to purchase more programming resources, should be directed to decision makers with the authority to approve financial requests.

- **Use several methods to convey the same evaluation results.** Depending on the diverse learning styles of stakeholders, different methods will be more or less effective with different types of people. Presenting the same results in more than one way will increase your chances of communicating effectively with all stakeholders.

- **Be honest and objective.** Try to recognize your own biases and take them into account when you are interpreting results. Do not exaggerate actual results in either direction. This is the most important guideline of all because if you are presenting inaccurate results, you might as well not be evaluating.

Recommended Standards

Standard	Rationale from Evaluation Results
Awareness/education programs	
• Achieve a 70% awareness level after six months of marketing and programming.	• Initial program indicated only 25% of first-time participants had a good understanding of specific programs.
• Attain an average attendance level of 60% in a seminar series.	• Attendance fluctuated greatly.

(continued)

Standard	Rationale from Evaluation Results
Evaluation/screening programs	
• Screen 80% of all employees in an annual cholesterol testing.	• Only 40% of all employees participated in the initial screening.
• Maintain a margin of error among skin fold testers within 3 mm per site.	• Individual body-fat readings varied greatly between annual HRA reports.
• All health fairs and screenings will be conducted in accordance with applicable laws and regulations.	• Federal legislation requires more clear-cut justification for wide-scale screening.
Staff	
• All staff are required to successfully complete a basic CPR course on a yearly basis.	• Two participants recently sustained minor injuries that required first aid.
• Screening staff must complete a training program in testing protocols and pass a practical exam.	• Health conditions reported by participants appear to be more varied each year.
• All teaching staff must complete a two-day training program in the content of each course they will teach and give a sample presentation.	• Participants have expressed concern about a lack of information provided in specific courses.
• Teaching staff must receive a score of 70% on the *Instructor Performance Form* before being assigned a class.	• More staff members are assuming teaching responsibilities.
Facility standards and customer service	
• No one waits at the reception counter for more than 15 seconds before being admitted.	• Suggestion box feedback suggests a lack of timely customer service at entry.
• No equipment will be down for more than 24 hours without an adequate written explanation for the members.	• Cardiovascular fitness areas are the most heavily used throughout the facility.
• New members receive a welcome letter within one month. Each member is greeted with a smile and is treated with courtesy and respect.	• Culture surveys indicate first-time participants are more likely to engage in multiple activities upon receiving their letter.

REVIEW QUESTIONS: APPLYING EVALUATION RESULTS

1. What types of guidelines would you follow to enhance the value of evaluation results?

2. Considering the varied learning styles of stakeholders, how would you attempt to effectively convey evaluation results to all parties?

3. Of the recommended standards previously listed, which ones do you feel would be most applicable at most worksites? And, what additional standards would you recommend for a typical worksite?

CHAPTER REVIEW

Summary

In order to prepare and present evaluation results that will be valued by key stakeholders, evaluators need to be objective as they interpret key data. In doing objective analysis, it is important to distinguish program significance from statistical significance, prepare appropriate data distributions, and identify key trends. Likewise, it is critical to identify key stakeholders to whom presentations and reports will be directed and to tailor these deliverables to their specific needs and interests. Evaluators should also be skilled in preparing appropriate graphs to clearly illustrate important facts and results that can be quickly understood by decision makers.

Overall, careful consideration should be given to various elements of the Socratic approach—who, what, where, when, why, and how—to ensure that stakeholders and decision makers can fully understand, use, and benefit from the evaluation results.

What Would You Do?

1. Your supervisor has recently requested that you review, analyze, and interpret participation and risk factor prevalence data on employees with the eventual goal of presenting your findings to various stakeholder groups. She has instructed you to format the printed (hard) copy for management with extensive narrative descriptions of the step-by-step process used to design and conduct the evaluation. You prepare a report consisting of 40% narrative and 60% graphic illustrations. Her response is critical, and she asks you to redo it with no more than two graphic illustrations. What reasons can you provide to support the idea that more than two graphic illustrations are needed?

2. You were recently promoted to health promotion evaluation analyst in a large managed care organization (MCO). One hundred of the MCO's corporate clients contract with your division for various health promotion services. Your responsibilities are to design, develop, and implement rigorous evaluations of these services. Evaluation reports will be tailored around the specific types of services provided to each client. Initially, you prepare a data collection planning framework similar to that shown in table 5.4 and submit it to your supervisor. She approves the framework and proposes a standard one-size-fits-all evaluation be developed for each client. Moreover, she indicates that each report should include a section focused on each type of data listed in the framework. You diplomatically respond by explaining that this is not feasible because WHP services are tailored about each client's individual request. In addition, you point out that all clients do not maintain databases for all data listed on the framework. She is perplexed to hear this and contends that any company interested in WHP should have these data on-site. You know otherwise, yet you want to tactfully demonstrate that all clients cannot be approached with the same level of expectation to produce the preceding data. What can you say to her to convey the need to approach each client individually? What would you do?

Appendix: Health Promotion and Evaluation Resources

Organization	E-mail address
Agency for Health Care Policy Research (AHCPR)	**www.ahcpr.gov**

AHCPR provides various data on state, regional, and national health care policies and cost-related statistics.

American Cancer Society (ACS)	**www.cancer.org**

ACS's Cancer Resource Center provides answers to questions about cancer, its causes, and its risk factors. You can find statistical information and links to other sites.

American College of Sports Medicine (ACSM)	**www.acsm.org**

One of America's premier research and certification organizations specializing in the field of exercise science.

American Health Care Association (AHCA)	**www.ahc.org**

AHCA's Health Services Research and Evaluation Group provides impact assessments of current and proposed public policy and provides statistics that describe the long-term health care developments. Various research reports and services are also available.

American Heart Association (AHA)	**www.americanheart.org**

AHA provides educational and research guides, programs, and resources. Its InfoGuide can be downloaded from its website.

American Hospital Association	**www.aha.org**

The American Hospital Association provides various educational and research publications for health care professionals working in health care settings.

American Lung Association (ALA)	**www.lungusa.org**

ALA provides various smoking cessation, asthma, and other respiratory health resources for worksite health professionals.

American Medical Association (AMA)	**www.ama-assn.org**

Medical claims data resources such as DRG and ICD software programs are available from AMA.

American Productivity and Quality Center (APQC)	**www.apqc.org**

APQC establishes benchmarking and best practices for worksite-based health and productivity management (HPM) programs.

American Public Health Association (APHA) www.apha.org

APHA is a national leader in a wide variety of public health areas and provides educational and research information and materials to organizations of all types.

American Psychological Association (APA) www.apa.org

APA provides access to information for consumers, the media, and worksite health professionals on depression and other mental health topics.

American Red Cross (ARC) www.redcross.org

The ARC provides first aid, CPR, and HIV/AIDS educational resources for worksite health professionals.

Association for Worksite Health Promotion (AWHP) www.awhp.org

AWHP provides worksite health professionals with print and electronic information on various employee health and productivity management topics.

Bureau of Labor Statistics (Department of Labor) www.bls.gov

BLS provides a wide array of data for use at the worksite about employee health, health care benefits, injury, and ergonomics.

Bureau of National Affairs, Inc. (BNA) www.bna.com

BNA is a major publisher of print and electronic news, analysis, and reference products spanning employee benefits, health care, and human resources.

Centers for Disease Control and Prevention (CDC) www.cdc.gov

CDC has many agencies that provide various scientific research on community and worksite health issues. The National Center for Health Statistics is a part of CDC.

Cooper Institute www.cooperinst.org

The Cooper Institute provides various training and certification programs, books, and services for health promotion and exercise science practitioners.

Crawford and Company www.crawfordandcompany.com

Crawford provides individual services as well as integrated claims and risk programs in various areas including workers' compensation and risk management.

Department of Health and Human Services (HHS) www.dhhs.gov

HHS contains numerous agencies that provide ready-to-use information on virtually any risk factor existing at the worksite.

Federal (USA) Statistics www.fedstats.gov

FedStats is a gateway to statistics from over 100 U.S. federal agencies.

Fitness Link www.fitnesslink.com

Fitness Link provides fitness and other health news items in addition to a free newsletter.

Fitness World   www.fitnessworld.com

Fitness World publishes newsletters, magazines, and other resources for fitness professionals to read and use in their purchasing decisions.

Health Care Financing Administration (HFCA)   www.hcfa.gov

HCFA administers Medicare, Medicaid, and other health insurance programs. Information on the Health Insurance Portability and Accountability Act (HIPAA) is available from HCFA.

International Health, Racquet   www.ihrsa.org
and Sportsclub Association (IHRSA)

IHRSA provides daily news clips on various corporate fitness issues and publishes various industry-related publications.

Managed Care Magazine   www.managedcaremag.com

This is a guide for managed care professionals covering capitation, compensation, disease management, NCQA, and HEDIS™.

Medline   www.nlm.nih.gov

This is housed within the National Library of Medicine and provides the latest health news around the world.

Mercer Company   www.mercer.com

Mercer is one of America's largest benefits consulting firms and publishes various health care economic data pertinent to employers.

Milliman and Robertson, Inc. (M&R)   www.milliman.com

M&R is one of the largest actuarial firms in the U.S. and provides various health care and employer-based medical data.

National Cancer Institute (NCI)   www.nci.nih.gov

NCI's Cancer Information Service is a good source for the latest, most accurate cancer information.

National Center for Health Statistics (NCHS)   www.cdc.gov/nchs

NCHS is part of the CDC and provides a huge inventory of national risk factor prevalence and cost data.

National Council on Compensation Insurance (NCCI) www.ncci.com

NCCI specializes in workers' compensation, injury, and ergonomic research.

National Heart, Lung   www.nhlbi.nih.gov/nhlbi
and Blood Institute (NHLBI)

NHLBI provides the latest research on heart, lung, and blood-related illnesses.

National Institute of Occupational Safety and Health (NIOSH)   www.cdc.gov/niosh

NIOSH is part of the CDC and specializes in occupational safety issues of all sorts.

Occupational Safety and Health Administration (OSHA)   www.osha.gov

OSHA is the nation's guardian of worksites and provides training resources as well as safety and ergonomic consultations.

Office of Disease Prevention and Health Promotion (ODPHP)   www.odphp.osophs.dhhs.gov

ODPHP provides the latest edition of Healthy People 2010 and other national health guidelines.

Society of Actuaries (SOA)   www.soa.org

SOA provides print and electronic resources on various types of medical care claims data.

Society for Prospective Medicine (SPM)   www.spm.org

SPM provides various print and electronic information on preventative medicine and health risk appraisals.

Wellness Councils of America (WELCOA)   www.welcoa.org

WELCOA provides a plethora of print and electronic health promotion resources for worksite health professionals. Topics ranges from back injury prevention to medical self-care.

Bibliography

American Productivity and Quality Center. 1998. *Health and productivity management: Consortium benchmarking study, best practice report*. Houston, TX: American Productivity and Quality Center.

Aquilina, D. 1990. How to formulate a data analysis strategy. *Business & Health* 8: 723-30.

Baun, W., W. Horton, and J. Storlie. 1992. *Guidelines for employee health promotion programs*. Champaign, IL: Human Kinetics.

Baun, W. and K. Wells. 1995. Evaluation processes steer Tenneco's health promotion program. *AWHP's Worksite Health* 1 (summer): 44-47.

Berkanovic, E., C. Telesky, and S. Reeder. 1981. Structural and social psychological factors in the decision to seek medical care for symptoms. *Medical Care* 29: 693-709.

Bernacki, E., S. Tsai, and S. Reedy. 1986. Analysis of a corporation's health care experience: Implications for cost containment and disease prevention. *Journal of Occupational Medicine* 28: 506-507.

Brady, W. and J. Bass. 1997. Defining total corporate health and safety costs—significance and impact: Review and recommendations. *Journal of Occupational and Environmental Medicine* 39: 224-231.

Broadhead, W.E., S. Gehlbach, F. DeGray, and B. Kaplan. 1989. Functional versus structural social support and health care utilization in a family medicine outpatient practice. *Medical Care* 27: 221-233.

Burton, W., S. Hutchinson, L. Helgesong, and J. Connor. 2000. An evaluation of a worksite prenatal education program: Five-year experience. *AWHP's Worksite Health* 6 (winter): 30-33.

Burton, W. and D. Conti. 1999. The real measure of productivity. *Business & Health* 17: 34-36.

Campbell, D. and J. Stanley. 1963. *Experimental and quasi-experimental designs*. Chicago: Rand McNally College.

Cascio, W. 1987. *Costing human resources: The financial impact of behavior in organizations*. 2d ed. Boston: PWS-Kent.

Chenoweth, D. 1998. *Worksite health promotion*. Champaign, IL: Human Kinetics.

Chenoweth, D. 1993. *Health care cost management: Strategies for employers*. Dubuque, IA: Brown & Benchmark.

Counte, M.A. and G.L. Glandon. 1991. A panel study of life stress, social support, and the health services utilization of older persons. *Medical Care* 29: 348-361.

Edington, D. and A. Braunstein. 1997. Ten research studies you can't afford to ignore. Parts III-V. *AWHP's Worksite Health* 3 (summer): 23-26; 4 (summer): 23-26; 5 (summer): 23-26.

Goetzel, R. and R. Ozminkowski. 1998. The relationship between modifiable health risks and health care expenditures. *Journal of Occupational and Environmental Medicine* 40: 843.

Hall, J. and J. Zwemer. 1979. *Prospective medicine*. Indianapolis: Methodist Hospital of Indiana.

Harris, J. 1992. *Managing employee health care costs: Assuring quality and value*. Beverly, MA: OEM Health.

Heaney, C. and R. Goetzel. 1997. A review of health-related outcomes of multi-component worksite health promotion programs. *American Journal of Health Promotion* 11: 290-308.

Hibbard, J. and E. Weeks. 1987. Consumerism in health care: Prevalence and predictors. *Medical Care* 25: 1019-1032.

Hunnicutt, D. and A. Deming. 1999. *Building a well workplace*. Vol. 1. Report. Omaha: Wellness Councils of America.

Kaman, R., ed. 1995. *Worksite health promotion economics*. Champaign, IL: Human Kinetics.

Kerlinger, F. 1973. *Foundations of behavioral research*. New York: Holt, Rinehart & Winston.

Kristein, M. 1997. Economic issues in prevention. *Preventive Medicine* 6: 252-264.

Lohr, K., R. Brook, and C. Kambery. 1986. Effect of cost-sharing on the probability of episodes of care for specific diseases. *Medical Care* 24, supplement: 18-30.

Lynch, W. and D. Vickery. 1993. The potential impact of health promotion on health care utilization: An introduction to demand. *American Journal of Health Promotion* 8: 89.

Lynch, W., H. Teitelman, and D. Main. 1991. The inadequacy of using means to compare medical costs of smokers and nonsmokers. *American Journal of Health Promotion* 6: 124-130.

McKenzie, J. and J. Smeltzer. 1997. *Planning, implementing, and evaluating health promotion programs: A primer*. 2d ed. Needham Heights, MA: Allyn & Bacon.

Milliman and Robertson. 1995. *Health risks and their impact on medical costs*. Milwaukee: Milliman and Robertson.

Murphy, R. 1987. Cost-benefit analysis in worksite health promotion evaluation. *Fitness in Business* 2: 15-19.

Naas, R. 1992. Health promotion programs yield long-term savings. *Business & Health* 10: 41-47.

National Institutes of Health. 1995. *NIH consensus statement*. Vol. 13. Bethesda, MD: National Institutes of Health.

Newkirk, J. 1998. Break into profit. *Fitness Management* 3 (March): 36-39.

Opatz, J., ed. 1994. *Economic impact of worksite health promotion*. Champaign, IL: Human Kinetics.

Opatz, J., ed. 1987. *Health promotion evaluation: Measuring the organizational impact*. Stevens Point, WI: National Wellness Association.

Oster, G., G. Colditz, and N. Kelly. 1984. *The economic cost of smoking and the benefits of quitting*. Lexington, MA: Heath.

Ostwald, S. 1986. Cost-benefit analysis. *AAOHN Journal* 34: 377-382.

Pelletier, K. 1996. A review and analysis of the health and cost-effective outcome studies of comprehensive health promotion and disease prevention programs: 1993-95 update. *American Journal of Health Promotion* 10: 380-388.

Pelletier, K. 1993. A review and analysis of the health and cost-effective outcome studies of comprehensive health promotion and disease prevention programs: 1991-93 update. *American Journal of Health Promotion* 8: 50-62.

Pelletier, K. 1991. A review and analysis of the health and cost-effective outcome studies of comprehensive health promotion and disease prevention programs. *American Journal of Health Promotion* 5: 311-315.

Peterson, J. 1991. Eight steps to making a successful presentation. *Fitness Management* 7 (July): 39.

Pronk, N. 1999. Relationships between modifiable health risks and short-term health care charges. *Journal of the American Medical Association* 282: 2235-2239.

Renwick, R., I. Brown, and M. Nagler, eds. 1996. *Quality of life in health promotion and rehabilitation*. Thousand Oaks, CA: Sage.

Rubinson, L. and J. Neutens. 1987. *Research techniques for the health sciences*. New York: Macmillan.

Ruchlin, H. and M. Alderman. 1980. Cost of hypertension control at the worksite. *Journal of Occupational Medicine* 22: 795-800.

Russell, L., M. Gold, and J. Siegal. 1996. The role of cost-effectiveness analysis in health and medicine. *Journal of the American Medical Association* 276: 1172-1177.

Stiglitz, J. 1988. *Economics of the public sector*. 2d ed. New York: Norton.

Suchman, E. 1967. *Evaluation research: Principles and practice in public service and social action programs*. New York: Russell Sage Foundation.

Vickery, D. 1996. Toward appropriate use of medical care. *Healthcare Forum Journal* 1 (January): 15-19.

Warner, K. 1993. The economic impact of worksite health promotion: Dollars and sense. *Action AWHP Newsletter* 1 (January/February): 1, 4.

Wilson, B. and T. Glaros. 1994. *Managing health promotion programs*. Champaign, IL: Human Kinetics.

Woodall, G., C. Higgins, J. Dunn, and T. Nicholsons. 1987. Characteristics of the frequent visitor to the industrial medical department and implications for health promotion. *Journal of Occupational Medicine* 29: 660-664.

Yandrick, R. 1996. *Behavioral risk management*. Tiburon, CA: Jossey-Bass.

Yen, L., D. Edington, and P. Witting. 1991. Associations between health risk appraisal scores and employee medical claims costs in a manufacturing company. *American Journal of Health Promotion* 6: 46-53.

Index

Note: Tables are indicated by an italicized *t* following the page number; figures by an italicized *f.*

A

A. Foster Higgins 91
absence frequency 19
absence rate 18
  absenteeism
  Bureau of Labor Statistics
    standards for 17-18
  case study 19
  data sources 91
  as dependent variable 17-19
  inconsistent definitions of 19
  as subjective or objective
    variable 16
absenteeism data, as evaluation
  tool 7
absolute-number-based variables
  148-149
abstract
  in reports 181
  sample of 181
accidents
  as common outcome 71
  data sources 91
  forecasting 82
  outcome variables 86
achievability, as goal criterion
  141, 143
adherence, defined 17
administrators, as stakeholders
  138-139
aggregate adjusted inflation rate
  124-125
aging population, as influential
  factor 83
American College of Sports
  Medicine 91
American Heart Association 60
American Hospital Association
  91
*American Journal of Health
  Promotion* 84
American Productivity and
  Quality Center 23
American Red Cross 91
analysis
  defined 33
  role in evaluation 34*f*
analytical process, of consultants
  58
ancillary resources, of consultants 60
annual reviews 10
anonymity, maintaining 184-185

appendixes, in reports 181
Association for Worksite
  Healthcare Promotion 91,
  177
attitudes/perceptions predictive
  factors 20*f*
attitudinal absence 19
audience, knowing 182, 185
audiovisual aids 183-184
automated recording, of productivity 25
average length of stay 69-70
awareness program standards
  186
AWHP's Worksite Health 84

B

Balke exercise stress test protocol
  37
Bank One Corporation 23, 24
baseline
  in absence of company data
    99-100
  in break-even analysis 106
  comparing data against 173
  for complex forecast 98-99
  for evaluations 167
  for simple forecast 98
  sources for 100
Behavior Risk Factor Surveillance System (BRFSS) 91
benefit-cost analysis
  about 118
  benefit-cost ratio method 120-
    121
  benefit identification and
    measurement 119
  comparison of costs and
    benefits 120-122
  cost identification and mea-
    surement 118-119
  as econometric tool 52
  in evaluation case study 150
  financial goal assessment 140
  in multiple interventions 121-
    122
  net benefit method 120
  as outcome evaluation tool 8
  present value *vs.* future value
    122-124, 125, 127
  sample framework 122*f*
  scenario 128

benefit-cost ratio method 120-
  121
benefit-cost ratios, declining 127*f*
benefit inflation 125
benefits
  defined 80
  planning factors 157*f*
  and present value adjustment
    126*f*
  terminology of 80
benefit variable
  break-even analysis calculation
    of 106-108
  defined 80
best case projections 86
bias
  self-selection bias 14
  subjectivity bias 42
  as threat to validity 41
blue-Monday absence 19
break-even analysis
  about 104
  baseline establishment 106
  benefit variable calculation
    106-108
  break-even point calculation
    108-109
  comparison of costs with and
    without intervention 107*t*,
    109*f*
  current benefit calculation 108
  as econometric tool 52
  financial goal assessment 140
  illustrating 182-183*f*
  penetration impact formula
    109-110
  preliminary steps for 104
  program-generated savings
    example 108*t*
  projected benefit calculation
    108
  sample cost-benefit
    comparison 105*f*
  sample six-month expense
    record form 105*f*, 106*f*
BRFSS (Behavior Risk Factor
  Surveillance System) 91
Bruce exercise stress test protocol
  37

budgetary pitfalls 14
Bureau of Labor Statistics
  absenteeism standards of 17-18
  as data source 91
  as index source 86
Bureau of National Affairs 91
Burton, Wayne N. 23-24
Business and Health 84, 100
business climate 14

C

cancer, as common outcome 71
carousel slide projector 183
case studies:
  absenteeism 19
  claims data analysis 56-57, 62-63
  control lack 27
  emergency department utilization 154
  evaluation design 157-158
  health care utilization 20-21
  low back injury prevention program 38-39
  risk factor cost appraisal 72-73
  stakeholders 139, 177-178
  trends 175
catastrophic events, as opportunity costs 119
Centers for Disease Control and Prevention 91
Ceridian Corporation 21
change rates, nominal *vs.* percentage graphs 84
Chrysler Corporation 21
Circulation 100
circulatory problems, as common outcome 71
claims data analysis
  about 52
  accessing and reviewing existing on-site claims reports 61-62
  additional data requests 64-65
  alternatives to in-house 57-60
  analysis goals development 63-64
  analyzing data 66-68
  applications of 52-53
  basic assessment 64
  beginning review 66
  case studies 56-57, 62-63
  classifying health care claim data 53-56
  common outcomes 71
  by consultants 57-58, 60
  grants for 60

health-related goal assessment 140
  in-house requirements 57
  by local resources 60
  as outcome evaluation tool 8
  phase 1 60-64
  phase 2 64-66
  phase 3 66-71
  practice analysis 68-70
  problem-focused questions 65
  questions formulation 64-65
  reporting conclusions 70-71
  step-by-step flowchart 59f
  suggested steps for 61
  trend identification 68
claims data report, sample 167t
clientele, of consultants 58
clinical/behavioral predictive factors 20f
comparison group 27
compensatory equalization of treatments 35
compensatory rivalry 35
complex forecast
  baseline for 98-99
  calculations for 101-102
  customized index 95f, 100f
  customized table 102f
  forecast data table 89-90
  indexes for 92-94
  influential factors 87-88
  selecting variable for 82
  time frame 88
complex variables 15
computer tips:
  database management software evaluation 33, 54
  evaluation goal development 168
  graph creation 183
  Internet searching 76
  matching groups variable selection 28
  program management software evaluation 6
  software-first approach 43
  spreadsheet calculation shortcuts 174
  spreadsheet computations 66
  spreadsheet software evaluation 113
conclusions, reporting 181
concurrent validity 41
confidentiality, maintaining 184-185
confounding variables 14-15

consultants
  claims data analysis by 57-58, 60
  indexes available from 86
consumer price index (CPI)
  caution in choosing 85
  as forecasting 81
content validity 41
Conti, Daniel J. 23-24
continuous quality improvement (CQI) 8
continuous trend sample 175f
contribution analysis 104. *See also* break-even analysis
control groups 26
control lack, case study 27
Corporate Monthly Report sample 180
cost
  of consultants 58
  and present value adjustment 126f
  terminology of 80-81
cost-avoidance benefits
  defined 80
  forecasting 103
cost data, on populations 172-174
cost distribution
  example graph 173f
  reporting 173
cost-effectiveness analysis
  about 110-111
  case study 114-115
  costing items in 112t
  as econometric tool 52
  example 5
  financial goal assessment 140
  forecasting value 115-117
  limitations 110-111
  as outcome evaluation tool 8
  performing 111-114
  sample framework 116f
  scenario 128
  smoking cessation intervention example 111t
  worksheet sample 115
  worksite back programs example 113f
cost information, separating by significant variables 173
cost item inflation 124
costs. *See* direct costs; fixed costs; health care costs; mixed costs; operational costs; opportunity costs; risk factor costs

cost-shifting, as influential factor 83
cost-volume-profit analysis 104. *See also* break-even analysis
couch potatoes 24
CPI (consumer price index). *See* consumer price index (CPI)
CQI (continuous quality improvement) 8
Crawford and Company 91
criterion-based validity 41
culture audit, data types 161*t*
customer service standards 187
customized indexes
 for complex forecast 95*f*, 100*f*
 data gathering and calculation 93-94
 selecting 85-86
 table for calculating 92

D

data
 accumulating over several years 65
 analysis and information 33-34, 34*f*
 chronological analysis 66-67
 comparing against reliable baseline 173
 consistency of 98
 defined 33
 degree of change in 98
 descriptive *vs.* inferential 161
 ensuring validity of 35-40
 on external populations 65
 perceived validity of 98
 quantitative *vs.* qualitative 160
 relevant data in claim data analysis 66-68
 retrospective data 98
 selecting items to measure 161-162
 for trends 96*t*
 types necessary to evaluation 159-161
data analysis
 econometric tools 52
 non-econometric tools 52
 Socratic elements 159*t*
database management software
 consultants' use of 58
 evaluation of 33, 54
data collection
 as external operation 164-165
 as in-house operation 164-165
 object of collection 164
 persons to collect 164

sample medical care claims form 165*f*
sample planning worksheet to record forms 166*f*
scheduling 168
Socratic elements 159*t*
data-driven goals 63
data formats
 about 165-167
 incorrect 168
 third-party computerized resources 166-167
data management
 evaluation 158-168
 planning framework 159*t*
data monitoring, Socratic elements 159*t*
data needs, of consultants 58
data reporting, Socratic elements 159*t*
data reviews, case study 34-35
data sources, questions for 162-163
data types, probable sources of 161*t*
decision makers
 financial goals of 140
 giving advance information to 184
 recommendations within power of 186
 as stakeholders 138-139
decision making
 evaluation's enhancement of 4
 and financial evaluation 5
demographic predictive factors 20*f*
demoralization of respondents 36
Department of Health and Human Services
 as data source 91
 major diagnostic categories 54
 risk factor status 73
dependent variables
 about 14
 absenteeism as 17-19
 health care utilization as 20
 participation as 17
 productivity as 23-26
 risk factor status as 21-23
 subclassifications of 15
descriptive data 161
diabetes
 baseline sources for 100
 and productivity loss 24
diagnostic related group (DRG)
 as health care claims data classification 54

and risk factor cost appraisal 73
sample inpatient claims and payments report 70*t*
diffusion of treatments 35
digestive disease 24
digestive problems, as common outcome 71
direct benefits, defined 80
direct costs
 defined 80
 examples of 118
direct observation, validity in 42
discount rate 123, 124-125. *See also* aggregate adjusted inflation rate
disease-prevention programs, expectations of 4
dollars, value of 122-124, 125, 127
double-barreled questions 41
downward trend 96*t*

E

econometric tools, data analysis 52
Edington, Dee 21
education program standards 186
emergency department utilization, case study 154
employee assistance programs (EAPs) 22
Employee Benefit Plan Review 84
Employee Benefits Research Institute 91
employee committee, as stakeholders 179
employee health, as quantitative data 161*t*
employees, incurring low or no costs 173
employee satisfaction, measuring 9
end-of-program outcomes, determining 5
enrollee subgroup composition 64
environmental assessment, data types 161*t*
environmental exposures, and risk factor status 22, 73
equipment
 in cost-effectiveness analysis 112*t*
 replacement costs 86
 resource identification 146

evaluation
  about 134
  baseline for 167
  case study 150
  communication flowchart
    sample 179*f*
  data management 158-168
  data types necessary to 159-
    161
  definition of 4
  financial 5, 6, 7
  history and maturity of
    program being evaluated
    139
  management reports 178
  political realities surrounding
    139
  program standards 187
  purpose of 4-5, 155
  rationale for 139
  time frame for 150-153.*See also*
    timing of evaluation
evaluation categories
  information use 6-8
  qualitative *vs.* quantitative
    issues 6
  summary of 10
  timing of evaluation 8-11
evaluation data, presenting 183
evaluation design, case study
  157-158
evaluation goals
  about 135
  data management 158-168
  design of evaluation 155-158
  evaluation resource identifica-
    tion 146-148, 156
  financial goals 140
  goal criteria 141-143
  health-related goals 140
  measurable objectives 143-145
  samples, with appropriate
    designs and tools 156*t*
  scenarios 138, 170
  scope of evaluation 148-153,
    154
  specificity of evaluation 153-
    154
  stakeholder identification 138-
    140
Evaluation Resource Assessment
  Grid 147
evaluation results
  applying 186-187
  conveying by several methods
    186
  interpreting 172-177
  reporting 179-185

ex ante benefit-cost analysis 118,
  119
executive summary, in reports
  181
expectancy effect 39
expense, by claim type 65
experimental designs
  about 29
  post-test only design 29*f*, 30
  pretest-post-test design 29
  staggered treatment design
    29*f*, 30-31
  time series design 29*f*, 30
experimental groups 26
ex post facto benefit-cost analysis
  118, 119
external data collection 164-165
external observation, of productivity 25
external populations 65
external validity
  defined 38
  reducing threats to 40
  threats to 39-40

F

facilities
  in cost-effectiveness analysis
    112*t*
  resource identification 146
  standards for 187
factors influencing health status
  (FIHS) 71
50th percentile 96
final report, of consultants 60
financial evaluation
  and decision making 5
  and process evaluation 7
  as quantitative issue 6
financial predictive facts 20*f*
financial resources, identifying
  146
First Card 24
fitness facility use, forecasting
  82
fixed costs, defined 80
forecast data table
  basic format 89*f*
  complex forecast 89-90
  simple forecast 89, 90*f*
forecasting. *See also* break-even
  analysis
  about 81
  blueprint of 88
  calculations 100-102
  comparison of costs with and
    without intervention 103*t*
  consistency of data 98
  cost-avoidance benefits 103

with cost-effectiveness analysis
  115-117
customized forecast data table
  88-90
customized indexes *vs.* standard indexes 85-86
data for indexes and baseline
  90-94
data sources 91
degree of change in data 98
as econometric tool 52
financial goal assessment 140
indexes and influential factors,
  sample indexes 86-88
influential factor determination
  83-84
key procedures 81
measurable variable selection
  82
perceived validity of data 98
periodicals as sources 84
philosophy and goals 98
recording results 100-102
representative forecast baseline
  94-100
retrospective data available
  98
time frame establishment 88
funding, compliance with
  specifications 5
future value *vs.* present value
  122-124, 125, 127

G

*General Evaluation Planning
  Checksheet* 134, 136
genetics, and risk factor status
  22, 73
goal criteria 141-143
goals. *See also* evaluation goals
  criteria for 141-143
  data-driven 63
  health-related goals 140
  reporting goals not met 178
graduated evaluation 129
graphs
  creating 183
  example of 184*f*
Great American Smokeout 40
group comparison
  about 26
  experimental and control
    groups 26
  matching groups 27-28

H

hard-copy program effectiveness
  reports 180-181
Hawthorne effect 39, 42

health care claims data classification
  by diagnostic related group (DRG) 54
  by international classification of disease (ICD) 53
  by major diagnostic category (MDC) 53
health care claims data reports 7
health care costs
  forecasting 82
  per risk factor 22*f*
  and risk factor status 21
health care delivery, and risk factor status 22, 73
Health Care Financing Administration
  as data source 91
  as index source 86
  major diagnostic categories 54
health care inflation, projecting 86
Healthcare Informatics 84
health care utilization
  case study 20-21
  data sources 91
  as dependent variable 20
  forecasting 82
  predictors by relative degree of influence 20*f*
health levels, factors influencing 65
Health Management Associates 74*f*
health-promotion programs, expectations of 4
health-related goals 140
health risk appraisals (HRAs)
  commercial analysis 43
  data entry 43
  data format issues 165
  employee feedback from 76-77
  as evaluation tool 7
  at First Card 24
  in-house analysis 43
  sample formats 43*f*
  types of 43
health risks, and productivity 24
heredity, and risk factor status 22
history
  as threat to internal validity 35, 37
  and treatment 40
HRAs (health risk appraisals). *See* health risk appraisals (HRAs)
hypertension, baseline sources for 100

I
ICD (international classification of disease). *See* international classification of disease (ICD)
imitation of treatments 35
impact evaluation 7, 10, 53
improper planning, as opportunity cost 119
inaccurate projections, as opportunity costs 119
inappropriate sampling 40
incidence rate, absenteeism 18
inclement weather 14
independent variables
  interventions as 14
  subclassifications of 15
indirect benefits, defined 80
indirect costs
  defined 80
  examples of 118
individual differences, hidden by total costs 173
industry norm 86
inferential data 161
inflation
  aggregate adjusted inflation rate 124-125
  data sources for rates 91
  medical inflation as influential factor 83
  projecting health care inflation 86
influential factors
  complex forecast 87-88
  determining 83-84
  simple forecast 87
information, defined 33
information use
  about 6
  impact evaluation 7
  outcome evaluation 7-8
  process evaluation 6-7
  summary of 10
in-house claims data analysis requirements 57
in-house data collection 164-165
injuries
  as common outcome 71
  data sources 91
  forecasting 82
  outcome variables 86
inpatient issues *vs.* outpatient issues 64-65
instrumentation
  invalid instrumentation 37
  as threat to internal validity 35, 37-38

intermediate evaluation time frame 151, 152*t*
intermediate-term trends 176
internal tracking systems, productivity 25
internal validity
  defined 35
  ruling out threats to 37-38
  threats to 35-37
international classification of disease (ICD)
  about 55
  data source issues 162-163
  as health care claims data classification 53
  inpatient claims report sample classification 55*t*
  outpatient claims report sample classification 55*t*
  and risk factor cost appraisal 73-77
  sample outpatient claims report 70*t*
International Health, Racquet and Sportsclub Association 91
International Quality and Productivity Center 91
Internet
  purchasing on as influential factor 83
  searching on 76
interventions
  and cost-effectiveness analysis 110-111
  as independent variables 14
  time frame as goal criterion 141, 143
introduction, in reports 181

J
Journal of Occupational & Environmental Medicine 84, 100
Journal of the American Heart Association 100
Journal of the American Medical Association 100

K
Kimberly-Clark Corporation 21
kurtosis, of trends 176

L
LCD projector 183
legislation, as influential factor 83
lifestyle behavior, and risk factor status 22, 73
limited discounts options, as influential factor 83

longitudinal data analysis 10, 11
long-range objectives 144
long-term evaluation time frame 151, 152*t*
long-term trends 177
low back injury prevention program, case study 38-39

M

major diagnostic category (MDC)
about 54
changes in various costs 67
data source issues 162-163
group summary of claims and payments example 69*t*
as health care claims data classification 53
outpatient claims and charges example 67*t*
and risk factor cost appraisal 73-77
standard MDCs 54-55
utilization ranking 66-67
male reproductive problems, as common outcome 71
management, reporting results to 178
Marion Merrill Dow 91
matching groups 27-28
materials
in cost-effectiveness analysis 112*t*
organizing for presentation 183
resource identification 146
maturation
interaction with selection 36
as threat to internal validity 35-36
mean
computing 97
interpreting with caution 173
vs. median 174*t*
measurability, as goal criterion 141, 142
measurement
defined 33
instruments for qualitative data 40-41
role in evaluation 34*f*
scheduling 152-153
Mecklenburg County Health Department 60
median
comparing 173
computing 96
using 97-98
vs. mean 174*t*
medical absence 19

medical claims, as quantitative data 161*t*
medical delivery, and risk factor status 22
medical inflation, as influential factor 83
Medicare, as influential factor 83
Medicine & Science in Sports & Exercise 100
MEDSTAT Group 23
mental health disorders 24
mental health programs 22
mental problems, as common outcome 71
methodology, in reports 181
migration, forecasting 82
Milliman and Robertson 86, 91
mixed costs, defined 81
mode, computing 97
monthly reviews 9
morbidity predictive factors 20*f*
mortality, defined 36
musculoskeletal problems, as common outcome 71

N

National Council on Compensation Insurance 91
National Health and Nutrition Evaluation Survey (NHANES) 91
National Institute of Occupational Safety & Health 91
negative information
reporting 178
value of 185
neoplasm, as common outcome 71
net benefit method 120
New York State Physical Activity Coalition 60
NHANES (National Health and Nutrition Evaluation Survey) 91
no change trend 96*t*
nominal changes *vs.* percentage changes 84*f*
non-econometric tools, data analysis 52
nonequivalent control group 27
non-experimental designs
about 32-33
pretest-post-test design 32*f*
time series design 32*f*

O

obesity, baseline sources for 100
objectives
approach to developing 145
establishing 143-145

objective variables 15-17
occupational injury reports 7
Occupational Safety and Health Administration 91
one group pretest-post-test design 32
on-site claims reports, accessing and reviewing existing 61-62
open-ended questions 41-42
operational costs, defined 81
opportunity benefits 80. *See also* indirect benefits, defined
opportunity costs
defined 81
examples of 119
oral reports 181-184
outcome evaluation
about 7-8
in claims data analysis 53, 71
sample factors in 10
outcomes
determining 5
reporting 181
outcome variables
affected by short-term interventions 149*t*
determining appropriate range of 148-149
equipment replacement costs 86
in evaluation case study 150
fitness center participation 86
health-related lost productivity 90*f*, 92*f*
injuries and accidents 86
low back injury cost 90*f*
risk factor incidence 86
specificity level 154
outpatient issues *vs.* inpatient issues 64-65
outside claims data analysis requirements 57-60
overhead transparency projector 183

P

participation
data sources for rates 91
as dependent variable 17
forecasting 82
outcome variables 86
penetration, defined 17
penetration impact formula 109-110
percentage changes *vs.* nominal changes 84*f*
performance indicators 121
periodic reviews
about 8

monthly, quarterly, semi-
annual, and annual reviews
9-10
quality assurance 8-9
summary of 10
personnel
competencies of 14
of consultants 58
in cost-effectiveness analysis
112*t*
resource identification 146
physical inactivity, baseline
sources for 100
placebo effect 39
planned absences 19
Planning Form for Goal Assessment
135, 137
poisoning, as common outcome
71
policies, changing 14
political realities 139, 184-185
populations, cost data on 172-174
post-test only design 29*f*, 30
predictive validity 41
presentations
deciding what to include in
183
identifying purpose of 181-182
presenteeism, measuring 24
present value adjustment 123-
124, 125, 126*f*, 127
present value *vs.* future value
122-124, 125, 127
pretest-post-test design 29, 31,
32*f*, 38
privacy, maintaining 184-185
problem-focused questions 65
problems, identifying 178
process evaluation 6-7, 10, 53
processing time, of consultants
58, 60
productivity
data sources 91
as dependent variable 23-26
forecasting 82
monitoring 39-40
obtaining valid measures of 25
relationship with specific
intervention 25
and risk factor status 21
productivity reports 7
program effectiveness designs
about 28
experimental designs 29-31
non-experimental designs 32-
33
quasi-experimental designs
31-32

program effectiveness reports
180-181
program management software,
evaluating 6
program objectives
approach to developing 145
establishing 143-145
program participants, as stakeholders 138, 179
program participation. *See*
participation
programs
comparison of 5
informing key groups about 5
program significance 172
progress, appraising 5
progress reports 180
project effectiveness evaluation,
as qualitative issue 6, 10
projectors 183
proportionate risk factor cost
appraisal technique (PRFCA)
73-77, 74*f*, 75*f*
Pygmalion effect 39

Q
Quaker Oats Company 21
qualitative-based productivity
outcomes 25
qualitative data
analyzing 42-45
designing instruments for
gathering 40-41
vs. quantitative data 160
qualitative issues
in process evaluation 6-7
vs. quantitative issues 6, 10
quality assurance
by consultants 58
in periodic reviews 8-9
quality reports 7
quantifiability, as goal criterion
141, 142
quantitative-based productivity
outcomes 25
quantitative data, *vs.* qualitative
data 160
quantitative issues *vs.* qualitative
issues 6, 10
quarterly reviews 9-10
quasi-experimental designs
about 31
pretest-post-test design 31
time series design 31*f*, 32
questionnaires 7
questions, types to avoid 41-42

R
rate-based variables 149

realistic achievability, as goal
criterion 141, 143
recommendations
based on specific results 186
within power of decision
makers 186
in reports 181
references, in reports 181
regional medical inflation 86
regression 36-37
relationships, in database
management software 54
relevant data, claim data analysis
66-68
reports
final report, of consultants
60
oral reports 181-184
politics of 184-185
program effectiveness reports
180-181
progress reports 180
scenario 188
written reports 179-181
resentful demoralization of
respondents 36
resource identification 146-148
resource redistribution, as
opportunity costs 119
result interpretation
cost data on populations 172-
174
program significance *vs.*
statistical significance 172
trend identification 174-177
results, reporting 181
retail medical inflation 86
return on investment ratio (ROI)
126*f*, 127
risk factor cost appraisal
about 52, 72
case study 72-73
economic significance of risk
factors 72
health-related goal assessment
140
proportionate risk factor cost
appraisal technique
(PRFCA) 73-77, 74*f*, 75*f*
scenario 78
risk factor costs, median annual
per employee 23*f*
risk factor incidence 86
risk factors
data sources 91
days lost per employee example 99*t*
defined 72

risk factors *(continued)*
   dollar value of productivity
      lost example 99*t*
   economic significance of 72
   rankings examples 72
risk factor status
   as dependent variable 21-23
   and health care costs 21
   influences on 22, 73
   national norms as average cost
      per risk 22
   and productivity 21
roller-coaster phenomenon 88

S

safety, as quantitative data 161*t*
scanners 43
scanning software 43
scenarios:
   benefit-cost analysis 128
   cost-effectiveness analysis 128
   evaluation goals 138, 170
   evaluation reports 188
   graduated evaluation 129
   graphic illustrations 188
   health promotion program
      evaluations 46-47
   program effectiveness evalua-
      tion 11
   risk factor cost appraisal 78
scheduled absences 19
scheduling
   for data acquisition 168
   in evaluation planning 146,
      148
   measurement 152-153
scope, of evaluation 148-153, 154
screening program standards
   187
selection
   interaction with maturation 36
   as threat to internal validity 36
   and treatment 40
self-reported feedback, of
      productivity 25
self-report instruments, validity
      in 41-42
self-selection bias 14, 19
semiannual reviews 9-10
sentinel effect
   about 39-40
   and direct observation 42
   as influential factor 83
setting, and treatment 40
severity rate, absenteeism 18, 19
shadow-pricing, as influential
      factor 83
short-term evaluation time frame
   151, 152*t*

short-term objectives 144
short-term trends 176
simple forecast
   baseline for 98
   calculations for 100-101
   customized table 101*f*
   forecast data table 89, 90*f*
   influential factors 87
   selecting variable for 82
   time frame 88
simple variables 15
skewness, of trends 176
slide projector 183
smokers 24
smoking cessation programs 40,
   110-111
social desirability effect 40
Society of Actuaries 91
Society of Prospective Medicine
   91
Socratic elements, data reporting
   and monitoring 159*t*
software evaluation
   database management soft-
      ware 33, 54
   with evaluation goals in mind
      168
   program management soft-
      ware 6
   spreadsheet software 113
sponsors, as stakeholders 138
spreadsheets
   calculation shortcuts 174
   computations 66
   evaluation of software 113
staff members
   performance standards for 9
   as stakeholders 138
   standards for 187
staggered treatment design 29*f*,
   30-31
stakeholders
   case study 139, 177-178
   goal criteria compatibility 141,
      142
   identifying 70, 138-140, 177
   management as 178
   needs of 177-179
standards, recommended 186-187
statistical regression 36
statistical significance 172, 174
stress management programs 22
subjective variables 16-17
subjectivity bias 42
support, change in source of 14
survey, of stakeholders 139-140

T

table of contents, in reports 181

tabulation, of surveys 45*f*
tabulation sheet sample 169*f*
tangible benefits, defined 80. *See
   also* benefit variable, defined
technology, as influential factor
   83
terminology
   benefits 80
   costs 80-81
   economic *vs.* econometric 52
testing, as threat to internal
   validity 37
time frame
   complex forecast 88
   for evaluation 150-153
   simple forecast 88
time series design 29*f*, 30, 31*f*, 32,
   32*f*
timing of evaluation
   longitudinal data analysis 11
   periodic reviews 8-10
   summary of 10
total quality management (TQM)
   8
treatments, diffusion of 35
trends
   case study 175
   continuous trend sample 175*f*
   data for 96*t*
   development rates for different
      types of variables 176
   identifying 68, 174-177
   kurtosis of 176
   skewness of 176
   time frames for 176
   variable trending patterns 175,
      176*f*
turnover patterns, forecasting 82
two-part questions 41
typical case projections 86

U

unplanned absences 19
unscheduled absences 19
unstructured questions 41-42
upward trend 96*t*
U.S. Department of Health and
   Human Services. *See* Department of Health and Human
   Services
utilization, defined 17

V

validity
   concurrent validity 41
   content validity 41
   criterion-based validity 41
   of data 35-40
   in direct observation 42

predictive validity 41
  in self-report instruments 41-42
value
  of dollars 122-124, 125, 127
  forecasting 115-117
variable costs, defined 80
variables
  about 14-15
  absenteeism as dependent
    variable 17-19
  absolute number based 148-
    149
  objective *vs.* subjective vari-
    ables 15-17
  participation as dependent
    variable 17
  productivity as dependent
    variable 23-26

rate based 149
risk factor status as dependent
    variable 21-23
  selected, for forecasting 82
  simple *vs.* complex variables 15
variable trending patterns 175,
    176*f*
varying standards, as influential
    factor 83
videocassette player 183

W

Watson Wyatt consultants 86
wholesale medical inflation 86
wide-scale evaluations 153
William Mercer, Inc. 86, 91
worker productivity index (WPI)
    23-24

workers' compensation
  data sources 91
  as quantitative data
    161*t*
Workers' Compensation
  Research Institute 91
workforce size, as influential
    factor 83
Worksite Environment Survey
    43, 44*f*, 45
Worksite Health Promotion
  (Chenoweth) 134
worktime, in cost-effectiveness
  analysis 112*t*
worst case projections 86,
    98
worst-day absence 19
written reports 179-181

About the Author

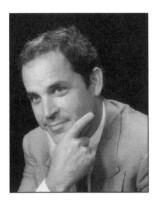

David Chenoweth, PhD, is a professor of health education and worksite health promotion studies at East Carolina University where he has taught evaluation courses for more than 20 years. Dr. Chenoweth has directed and conducted evaluation projects in the public and private sectors for over two decades as president of Health Management Associates. He's made more than 400 presentations to various business and health care groups and has authored seven books, including *Planning Health Promotion at the Worksite*, *Health Care Cost Management*, and *Worksite Health Promotion*.

He is a fellow of the Association for Worksite Health Promotion (AWHP) and first vice president of AWHP's education committee. He received his PhD from The Ohio State University in 1980.

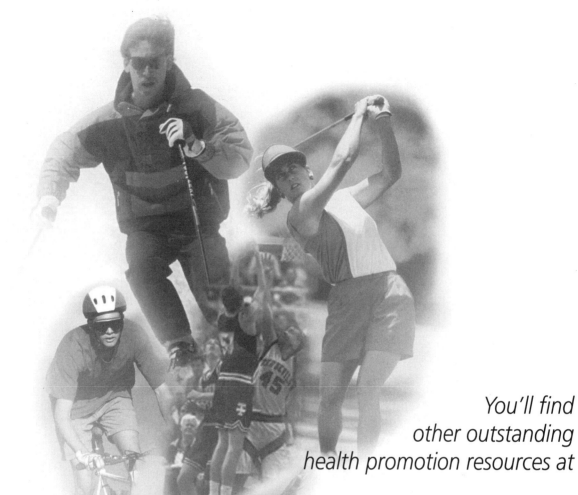